IS YOUR CHILD *ALLERGIC?*

Common-sense, practical information about childhood allergies, their causes and treatment especially written for parents by a specialist consultant paediatrician.

GW00391750

IS YOUR CHILD

ALLERGIC?

A Practical Guide for Parents

Jan A. Kuzemko
MD, FRCP, DCH

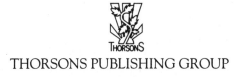

THORSONS PUBLISHING GROUP

First published in 1988

© JAN KUZEMKO 1988

All rights reserved. No part of this book may be reproduced or utilized in any form or by any means, electronic or mechanical, including photocopying, recording or by any information storage and retrieval system, without permission in writing from the publisher.

British Library Cataloguing in Publication Data

Kuzemko, Jan A.
Is your child allergic?: a practical guide for
parents.
1. Pediatric allergy
I. Title
618.92'97   RJ386

ISBN 0-7225-1434-4

Cover illustration by Jane Hiffey

Published by Thorsons Publishers Limited,
Wellingborough, Northamptonshire, NN8 2RQ,
England.

Printed in Great Britain by Woolnough Bookbinding Limited,
Irthlingborough, Northamptonshire.

5   7   9   10   8   6   4

Contents

	Introduction	7
Chapter 1	A Brief History of Allergy	9
Chapter 2	The Causes of Allergy in Children	12
Chapter 3	What Is Allergy?	20
Chapter 4	The Genetic and Environmental Factors in Allergy	29
Chapter 5	How Common Are Allergies in Children?	31
Chapter 6	Food Allergy	39
Chapter 7	Skin Allergies	66
Chapter 8	Allergies of the Nose	81
Chapter 9	Allergies of the Ears	93
Chapter 10	Allergies of the Eyes	97
Chapter 11	Asthma	100
Chapter 12	Anaphylaxis	128
Chapter 13	Allergies to Bites and Stings	131
Chapter 14	Reactions to Drugs and Medications	135
	Glossary	139
	Index	143

Dedication

I would like to thank Wendy Wilson, Senior Commissioning Editor, for helpful advice and support during the writing of this book.

Introduction

For many years, the parents of children with allergic disorders such as asthma, eczema, nasal and food problems, have sought my advice, or have written to me asking for factual information, about the management of their children's disorders. Although some knowledge about allergies in general is available in technical books, there is hardly any practical information about the allergies of infants and children written specially for the general reader.

This book describes all the common allergies of infants and children and is intended primarily for parents. Professionals and students in specialities allied to medicine or children's diseases will also find the book a useful source of objective information.

Chapter 1

A Brief History of Allergy

Allergic disorders have been affecting man since time immemorial. The Egyptian Ebers Papyrus, written around 1550 BC, gives a full description of asthma and its possible remedies. Even earlier — around 2640 BC — King Menes was depicted as having died following a wasp sting allergy. Hippocrates, 'The Father of Medicine' (460-350 BC), described in detail asthma in children, and pointed out that cold air could precipitate wheezing and cough. The exact way the inhalation of cold air causes asthma had to await the discoveries of the 1980s. Hippocrates also described allergy to cheese. Hay fever was known to Persian physicians of the eleventh century. The ancient Chinese practised inhalation of herbs in the treatment of asthma, and the Romans and Greeks in the second and third centuries AD associated some attacks of asthma with emotional factors, but progress in the understanding of allergies was fairly slow up to the eighteenth century when an Edinburgh physician, William Cullen, coined the word 'idiosyncrasy' when describing patients unable to tolerate milk, eggs and shellfish. There is little doubt that he was speaking about food allergy. Subsequently, British physicians such as John Bostock (1773-1845) and Charles Blackley (1820-1900), both hay fever sufferers themselves, finally proved by a series of meticulous experiments that grass pollens were responsible for the symptoms and signs of 'hay fever'. Leonard Noon and John Freeman in 1911 added further to our knowledge by showing that an injection of grass pollen extracts in water could alleviate the condition.

With the advent of microscopy in the late nineteenth century, scientists were given the opportunity to describe in detail the changes of various disease processes and make new observations. Paul Ehrlich (1854-1915) first described in 1878 the presence of the *mast cell* in the lung connective tissues and suggested that the cell might act as a storage cell. Fifty years later it was found that the mast cell was a potent source of many biological substances which were released during allergic reactions, thus pointing the way to the development of active treatments for allergy by preventing the release of these substances from the mast cells and hence preventing adverse allergic reactions occurring in the patients.

Von Pirquet and Bela Schick (1906) were two Viennese children's physicians who first suggested that the word 'allergy' should be given to an unusual phenomenon that they had observed in a small number of children. They noticed that some infants and children immunized for the second or third time against diphtheria developed, for some reasons which were most obscure, severe reactions characterized by a high fever, signs of shock, breathing problems, and leading occasionally to a fatal outcome. They postulated further that the first injection of diphtheria antitoxin 'changed or altered the child's body reactions to the subsequent injections'. Allergy comes from the Greek 'allos' (altered) and 'ergon' (reaction). Now we know that Von Pirquet and Schick were describing anaphylactic reactions (anaphylaxis means extreme sensitivity to an injected allergen, i.e. protein, following a previous injection) to the proteins of the horse sera which were employed at the time in immunization procedures.

A German researcher Carl Prausnitz (1876-1963), who was a hay fever sufferer, and Heinz Kustner (1897-1961), who was his patient and was allergic to fish, demonstrated that allergic sensitivity could be transferred from one individual to another. A small amount of Kustner's purified blood was injected into Prausnitz's left arm and 24 hours later an extract of fish was applied to his arm. Within minutes he developed a small area of itching, redness and swelling — i.e. a positive skin test. The discovery has been termed as the 'passive transfer test'.

During the 1920s two American physicians, Coca and Cooke, coined the term atopy (from Greek, meaning a strange disease) and suggested that the word be applied to those allergic disorders in humans which appeared to have a familial or hereditary basis such as asthma, hay fever and eczema. Since then atopy has acquired many different meanings. Some use it interchangeably with allergy and its various disorders such as food allergy, hyperactivity in children, etc. Others state that the term should be restricted to those conditions in which a reaginic antibody (IgE) is produced in response to the allergens in the environment.

During the 1960s a husband and wife team in the USA,

Kimishige and Teruko Ishizaka, isolated a component from allergic human blood that had completely different characteristics from any of the known protein fractions. Further investigations showed that this particular protein carried the reaginic activity associated with some allergic reactions. The World Health Organization (WHO) designated this new immunoglobulin class as 'IgE'. Utilizing these concepts, P.G.H. Gell and R.R.A. Coombs, two British immunologists, described a classification of allergic reactions which offered a rational understanding of the complex mechanisms involved. No doubt further detailed advances will occur in the years to come which will eventually explain the puzzles of allergy.

One of the earliest prescriptions for the treatment of asthma is found on the clay tablets of the Assyrians and Babylonians, about 2025 BC.

> 'If the patient is suffering from a wheezing cough . . . pound roses and mustard together, drop it in purified oil on to his tongue, also fill a tube with it and blow it into his nostrils.'

The mode of administration of this particular medication is very reminiscent of the 'modern' treatment of asthma where inhaled agents are used!

Chapter 2

The Causes of Allergy in Children

A large number of substances exist in the world which can be involved in allergic reactions. In general, these are proteins of some form, i.e. nitrogenous compounds that are essential constituents of all living organisms. Often the allergic reactions are fairly obvious — for instance, when a child develops recurrent itchy eyes and a runny nose during the pollen season. At other times the allergy-connection can be obscure unless a very exacting history is obtained, or some specialized investigations are carried out, or deliberate and laboratory controlled allergen challenges are carefully monitored. Moreover, at times symptoms and signs of a disease can be caused by a similar or even identical allergen which is present in an animal or its products, e.g. horse dander and horse serum (cross reactions).

The allergens to which an infant or child may become sensitive are:

Ingestants
Inhalants
Injectants
Physical agents
Contactants
Miscellaneous agents

INGESTANTS — FOOD ALLERGENS

The common food allergens are cow's milk, eggs, cereals, fish, nuts, spices, fruits, and some vegetables. It is worth remembering that some children can develop symptoms and signs not because they are allergic to a particular food but because the reactions have

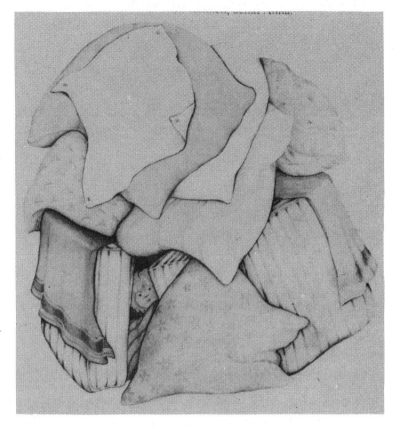

Figure 2.1   I am hiding from allergies!

resulted from toxicity, food additives and preservatives, bacterial or fungal contamination, or food intolerance. Many infants and children suffer from allergies to food but some do not — one must not jump to conclusions.

Jeremy was a perfectly normal boy at birth. His mother tried to breast feed him initially but developed a breast abscess and changed reluctantly to cow's milk feeds. Soon Jeremy started to develop recurrent bouts of watery diarrhoea, became thin, lost weight and grew apathetic. Professional advice suggested cow's milk allergy, hence Jeremy was commenced on a milk prepared from vegetable sources. He started to grow again and to thrive splendidly. At the age of one year attempts were made to introduce cow's milk again but the bouts of diarrhoea returned. A further attempt was made at the age of 18 months with similar adverse results. Specialized investigations at this stage revealed that Jeremy was born with an absent enzyme which is normally present in the digestive system and which helps to break down lactose, the sugar present in the milk. Thus, although Jeremy demonstrated features of allergy, he was not allergic to cow's milk but he could not digest the sugar present in the milk because he was lacking the specific digestive enzyme.

Nonetheless, the proteins in cow's milk are important allergens in infants. There are at least 50 such proteins in cow's milk, of which beta-lactoglobulin is the commonest. Human milk does not contain any beta-lactoglobulin. When cow's milk is boiled, some of these proteins are destroyed, but not all. Thus on rare occasions an infant will tolerate boiled or evaporated milk but not fresh cow's milk. In addition, some cow's milk proteins are found in beef and similar meat products. Thus a child experiencing symptoms eating beefburgers may, in fact, be allergic to these specific proteins rather than to other impure substances in meats, e.g. additives which can cause food induced illnesses not mediated by a known immunological mechanism.

The breast fed baby may be at risk of developing allergies as well. Some food allergens can pass to the foetus through the placenta and cause the baby in the womb to be sensitized to them. Once born, if the baby becomes exposed to similar allergens, a reaction may occur and cause symptoms. Other noxious agents such as insecticides and environmental contaminants can be absorbed by the mother in food and passed subsequently to the baby in the breast milk.

Egg white is a very potent sensitizer. It is doubtful whether sensitivity to pure egg yolk has ever been documented. An infant allergic to a chicken egg is usually sensitive to chicken meat. A thorough boiling of eggs will often destroy the proteins responsible for reactions. Since the egg white is widely used in various foodstuffs, it is essential to check their composition very carefully if allergy is suspected. In addition, vaccines are grown on chick embryos and are best avoided in children allergic to chicken eggs. At times the merest contact with an allergen in an already sensitive child can result in severe symptoms, as illustrated in the following case history.

Mark, aged 9 years, had a long history of chicken egg sensitivity causing skin rashes and bouts of wheezing. His parents diligently avoided chicken eggs and foodstuffs containing egg white so that he has remained in good health for many months. One day his mother took him to the local market where she got involved in a conversation with a passing acquaintance. Mark, who became progressively more bored throughout these proceedings, started to touch the stall on which eggs were placed. Within minutes he developed an intense and generalized itching rash and swelling of lips, face and hands after touching the eggs. He required urgent hospital treatment.

Comment: Although foods usually have to be eaten to cause symptoms and signs, in a sensitive child contact with a food can cause reactions. A similar example occurred in a little girl allergic to fish who developed a sudden attack of asthma after inhaling fish odour in a restaurant. But it is not all gloom — a child allergic to cod fish will, as a rule, tolerate cod liver oil!

Wheat is the main allergen of cereals. Wheat flour is used in the making of bread, pasta, etc. In my experience, rice (especially polished rice) is rarely responsible for adverse reactions. This is because the allergens in rice are present in the rice hull, i.e. the outer covering of the rice grain which is removed in making polished rice.

Nuts are strong allergens. They are found throughout the world and are used extensively in confectionery. The reactions tend to be severe and are often to a particular type of nut, e.g. peanuts. However, some children allergic to alder, birch, or hazel tree pollens can produce reactions if they eat hazel nuts and occasionally apples or other similar fruits. Almonds, which contain 40-60 per cent oil, are used in cosmetics and flavours, and are potent allergens.

Fruit and vegetables cause reactions occasionally. Potatoes are rarely responsible for allergic reactions except in those tree pollen allergic children who while helping their mothers may develop skin rashes, nasal symptoms and itchy and weepy eyes. There is some cross-reactivity between potatoes and tomatoes because they belong to the same botanical family. Oranges and orange juices contain various colours and aromatic agents which may be responsible for toxic reactions rather than causing true allergy.

INHALED SUBSTANCES

Inhaled allergens are absorbed through the lining membrane of the nose or the respiratory system which then act as the shock organs. At times the skin may be the shock organ so that when a child inhales an allergen to which s/he is sensitive acute skin rash or eczema will be produced rather than the expected reactions within the nose or the chest.

Allergens of practical importance are pollens, animal hair, dander and its skin sheddings, house dust, the house dust mite, feathers, and moulds and yeasts.

Plants pollinate by dispersing their pollens either by wind or by insects. The first group produces a huge number (even millions!) of tiny tough or dry male grains, whereas the second group yields smaller numbers of large and sticky substances. Thus it is the wind dispersed pollens which are largely responsible for clinical disorders in children, and on the whole they do not travel long distances before reaching ground level. Admittedly tree pollens can occasionally travel far — birch pollens from East Anglia have been recovered at sea about 30 kilometres from land — but this is an unusual observation.

There are thousands of species of grasses — indeed about 15 per cent of the world's surface is occupied by them and there is evidence that their territories are spreading, e.g. in areas of deforestation. However, only a small number such as cocksfoot, fescue, rye-grass, foxtail, timothy, and fog are of clinical importance. In Europe, the pollination period extends from May to August or early September. Weeds such as dandelion and plantain pollinate in short bursts during the spring and summer months.

Most trees produce large amounts of pollen but their flowering periods vary. Thus alder trees flower in early March/April and silver birch and beech around May time. Evergreen trees tend to produce huge amounts of pollens — the worst offenders are cedars, junipers and cypresses.

Animal hair, dander and its superficial skin sheddings are powerful allergens. Exposure may be due to the inhalation by the child of allergic particles which may come from the animal's skin, urine or saliva, and the allergic reactions may also occur through indirect contact with an animal — for example even wearing a dress or playing with a toy that had been in contact with an animal can occasionally cause severe reactions. The cat is probably the most allergenic animal ever tested, followed by the dog, probably

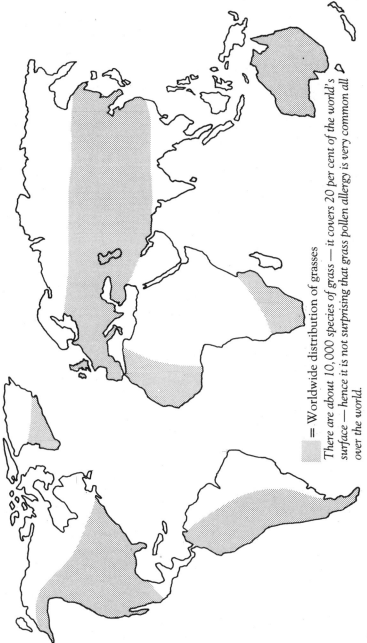

= Worldwide distribution of grasses

There are about 10,000 species of grass — it covers 20 per cent of the world's surface — hence it is not surprising that grass pollen allergy is very common all over the world.

Figure 2.2   Grasses in the World

because one of the proteins responsible for acute allergic reactions is similar in both species. The horse is a common source of severe allergy — often as a result of contact.

Allergy to house dust is common because the dust contains a mixture of organic matter, pollens, bacteria, insects, dander, mites etc. Pure preparations of dust act as irritants rather than cause allergic reactions. The house dust mite (life cycle of three months) is the most important allergen recovered from the house dust. They proliferate most when the temperature is about 25°C and in a relative humidity of 70 per cent or over, and because the mite obtains most of its nutrients from shed human skin scales it is most abundant in beds and bedrooms. Symptoms occur when the child inhales the excreta of house dust mites or their desiccated bodies.

Inhalation of mould spores is not uncommonly responsible for seasonal symptoms. Spores are smaller than the majority of pollens and are more plentiful — thus they are easier to inhale than pollen grains.

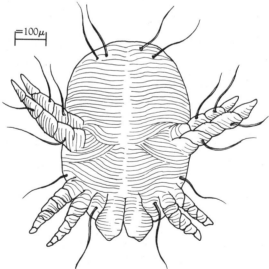

Figure 2.3   Microscopic view of the House Dust Mite

This is a female mite — DERMATOPHAGOIDES PTERONYSSINUS. Each mite produces over 10 waste particles in any 24 hours. Allergy is caused by proteins in the mite or the mite waste particles. These waste particles are extremely light and can float in the air, e.g. as when bedding is disturbed. The allergic child inhales the waste particles and thus develops symptoms of asthma. Each female mite can increase the mite population by about 30 every 20-30 days.

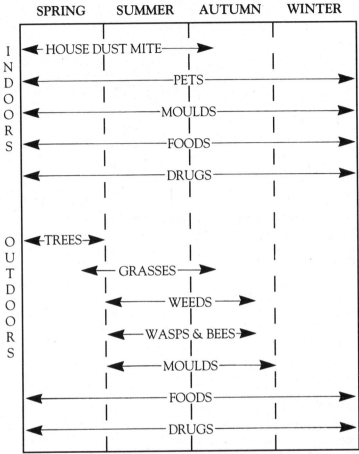

Figure 2.4   What type of allergies to expect and when

There are many other inhalant allergens to which the child can be exposed occasionally. Kapok hair is used in making cushions and sleeping bags; flax-seed is a component of some hair sprays and insulating materials; vegetable gums are used in large numbers of products such as hair sprays, cosmetics, paper making, foods such as chocolates and jelly beans, ice cream, etc.

Thus in all situations when the child is suspected of being allergic it is essential to obtain a detailed and comprehensive history, which can then lead to the confirmatory laboratory and clinical tests and offer a guide to an effective treatment of the allergic condition.

Chapter 3

What Is Allergy?

When a noxious organism or agent invades the human body, a series of defence mechanisms is immediately set into operation in order to protect the individual from possible harmful damage. This defence mechanism, which has the ability to recognize, 'remember' and deal with these various foreign components of the body, is termed the immune system. As a rule, the immune system recognizes and attacks the foreign matter but not the normal body constituents of the individual. However, occasionally, when things go wrong for some reason, the body can react against its own tissues and cause extensive damage to organs. This process is called *auto-immunity* and occurs, for instance, in children who develop a certain form of kidney disease or rheumatoid arthritis.

Similarly, the infant or the child who is allergic possesses an immune system that can be detrimental.as well. It synthesizes, or makes, specific 'protective' substances when exposed to an allergen — so-called immunoglobulin E, or for short, IgE antibodies. The allergic reaction happens when the child renews his/her contact with the same or similar allergen to which s/he has been previously exposed (i.e. sensitized) and the reaction results in the release of characteristic pharmacological substances (also called mediators) by certain specialized cells of the body causing specific and often reproducible signs and symptoms of a disease such as asthma, eczema or hay fever, etc. These reactions occur fairly quickly, i.e. within minutes, and they may give rise to other reactions within a few hours or even days.

The cells of the immune system, which are capable of recognizing and reacting in a specific way with the many thousands of different foreign protein substances, are called lymphocytes (from the Latin 'lymph' meaning water) and are specialized white blood cells. These cells are widely distributed in the body tissues such as the blood, the bone marrow, in the lymph

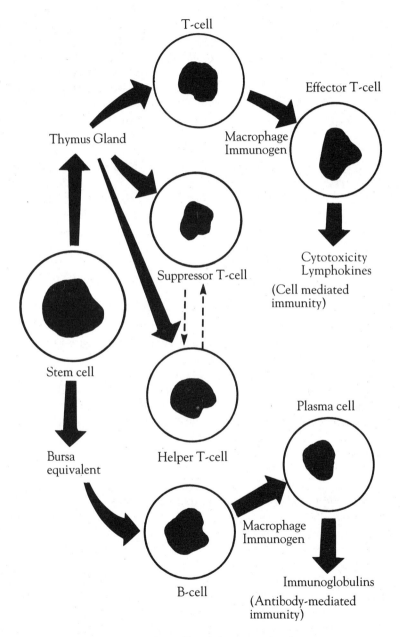

Figure 3.1   The cells of the Immune System

nodes and lymph tissues of the gastrointestinal tract. The immune system consists of two parts: the cell-mediated and the humoral parts (i.e. involving body fluids). The lymphocytes which involve the cell-mediated part are called T-lymphocytes because they mature in the thymus gland which is sited in the neck. They are predominantly active in killing viruses, parasites, moulds and are involved in the rejection of transplant organs. A subgroup of T-lymphocytes are called helper or supressor cells because they are capable of increasing and decreasing immunological reactions. The lymphocytes which take part in the humoral immunity are termed B-lymphocytes and their main function is to produce antibodies after contact with foreign protein, i.e. to make 'protective' immunoglobulins. The true origin of B-lymphocytes is not fully known — hence they have been named after the organ in birds where they were first identified — the bursa of Fabricius.

Not all foreign agents evoke similar immune responses in the child. Those which have the ability to react with antibodies are termed antigens or allergens — i.e. they stimulate the production of IgE antibodies (or reagins). It follows that these foreign substances must possess certain unique properties in order to make them either more or considerably less 'immunogenic' than other particles. In general, they are complex proteins and the reactions they may elicit will depend on the dose, the way they were absorbed (some substances can be tolerated if eaten but not when inhaled), the rate at which they had been taken, and importantly, on the genetic factors in the child.

The immunoglobulins (or antibodies) are synthesized by the B-lymphocytes and can be found extensively in almost all the body tissues and fluids such as sweat, blood, saliva, mother's milk, etc. They have similar basic structures and can bind (or attach themselves) in a specific way to the allergen. So far, five different classes of immunoglobulin have been discovered.

1. **IgG** — it accounts for 75 per cent of total immunoglobulins in the human blood and consists of four sub-classes.

IgG_1 — 60 to 70 per cent
IgG_2 — 15 to 20 per cent
IgG_3 — 4 to 8 per cent
IgG_4 — 2 to 6 per cent

It is the only immunoglobulin which crosses the placenta from the mother to the unborn baby. Hence, it affords protection against many infections when the baby is born. IgG_4 has been found to bind to the mast cells and is associated with some allergic reactions causing childhood asthma.

2. **IgA**—is most abundant in body tissues such as saliva, secretions from the airways and other mucous membranes. Can be passed from the mother to the baby in breast milk and affords local protection against various noxious organisms.

3. **IgM** — is involved in the various immune processes of the body but not in allergic reactions.

4. **IgD** — its function remains unknown.

5. **IgE** — blood concentrations in normal children are very low but rise in those with allergic disorders. It is believed that the original biological function of the IgE antibody was to protect the human against the invasion of parasitic infestations because the blood levels in children and adults harbouring parasites are very high indeed. In developed societies its importance lies in the causation of acute allergic reactions when the allergen comes into contact with the mast cell and some other special cells (basophils) which are already bound with IgE.

The specialized cells which synthesize IgE are located in the lymphoid tissues of the body, in the linings of the alimentary tract, and in the respiratory system. This synthesis of excessive production of IgE antibody is under genetic control and it depends on the complex interactions between the B- and T-lymphocytes and IgE antibodies. The newly born baby has almost undetectable IgE antibody levels in the blood stream. The levels increase gradually throughout infancy and childhood and reach adult levels by about 14 years of age. There is some evidence that high IgE levels in the blood taken from the umbilical cord immediately after the baby is born may predict whether the baby is at an increased risk of developing allergy within the first two years of life. This important finding, if confirmed by other studies, may be of great clinical importance as it may help in early diagnosis and management of some allergic disorders, and even their prevention by breast feeding or specialized diets. Breast feeding itself does not affect blood IgE levels.

IMMUNOLOGICAL MECHANISMS IN ALLERGIC DISORDERS

For practical purposes allergic reactions have been divided into four main groups. This classification is helpful in understanding the various types of reaction that may occur. It is realized however, that such a working scheme does not explain many other complex processes which may be involved in allergic reactions, and it is very likely that additional and unknown categories of reaction co-exist or occur.

Type I allergy or IgE mediated

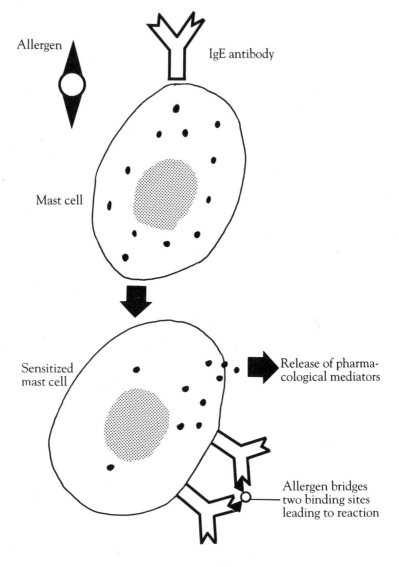

Figure 3.2   Type 1 Reaction

The allergy is caused by IgE antibodies, although other classes of immunoglobulins may be involved rarely. The specific IgE antibody attaches itself to the mast cell or the basophil (a circulating white blood cell so termed because it is easily stained by basic dyes). The mast cell in the human is found in the lungs, the upper respiratory tract, in the intestinal tract and in the skin. The mast cells contain granules of histamine and other active pharmacological substances which, when released from these cells, are capable of producing an acute allergic reaction and causing specific symptoms and signs, e.g. asthma. The symptoms appear very quickly, usually within ten minutes or so, hence the reaction is called the immediate type allergic reaction. Histamine is the most important agent released during such a reaction and it causes the blood vessels to dilate so that they become more permeable to the passage of tissue fluid out of the vessels, which leads to swelling formation, e.g. in the skin. In the lungs, histamine causes the swelling of the membrane lining the airways and the contraction of the special muscle which surrounds the airways. Hence it leads to narrowing of the breathing tubes and to excessive production of mucus in the airways making them even more narrow. Clinically, the child will develop difficulties with breathing and a repetitive cough so as to clear the airways and s/he will start to 'wheeze' — a musical noise which is produced when the air is expelled from the lungs through very narrow tubes — i.e. the signs of asthma appear. In the nose, the excessive amounts of mucus will cause its obstruction, swelling of the lining, itchiness and bouts of sneezing. In the skin, histamine produces redness and elevated patches which itch intensely. Histamine, one of the oldest discovered mediators of allergy, has been used here as an example, but there are other important agents which are also released during these reactions. The nature of some of these agents and their full relevance remains to be fully elucidated. Fig. 3.3 demonstrates diagrammatically the various processes of allergic reaction just described.

In some children the mast cells can be damaged not only by these immediate allergic reactions but also by non-allergic mechanisms, the nature of which remains obscure. But whatever the nature of the cell damage, the clinical symptoms and signs that ensue will always be similar, as for instance in those children who develop recurrent hives which can be caused by true allergy or food intolerances which are not associated with recognized immunological mechanisms.

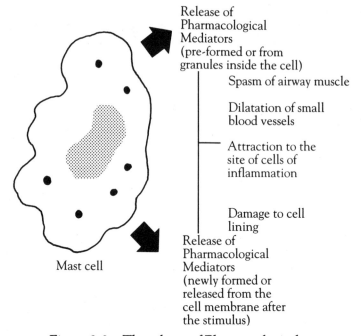

Release of
Pharmacological
Mediators
(pre-formed or from
granules inside the cell)

Spasm of airway muscle

Dilatation of small
blood vessels

Attraction to the
site of cells of
inflammation

Damage to cell
lining

Release of
Pharmacological
Mediators
(newly formed or
released from the
cell membrane after
the stimulus)

Mast cell

**Figure 3.3   The release of Pharmacological
Mediators from the Mast Cell**

Type 2 reactions

Here the antibodies circulate freely while the allergen is attached
to membranes of certain types of cell. When the allergen and the
antibodies react together, a number of reactions occur and involve
various other 'protective' proteins—(one of these is called
complement). These processes lead to the damage of the cells and
they vary in the rapidity of onset. Some childhood anaemias
where the red blood cells are rapidly destroyed is one example.

Type 3 reactions

These are complex reactions. They involve freely circulating
antibodies, which usually belong to the IgG class, and the
complement and the local accumulation of allergen. A so-called
complex is formed (of allergens or antigens and antibodies) which
is responsible for the tissue damage. Serum sickness is a historical
and classic example of Type 3 reaction. Here a foreign animal
protein is introduced to the human. Thus the synthesis of
antibodies is rapidly induced and the antigen-antibody complexes
are formed which deposit themselves in various tissues of the body

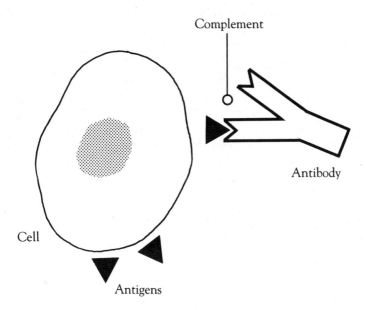

Figure 3.4   Type 2 Reaction

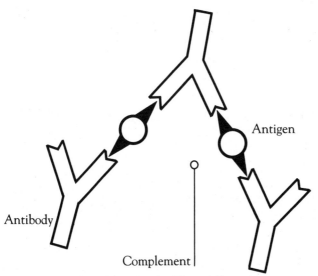

Figure 3.5   Type 3 Reaction

causing severe and extensive cell damage. Some observations suggest that this particular reaction may be involved in some cases of food allergy.

Type 4 reactions

In these reactions antibodies are not involved. The reactions are mediated by thymus-derived lymphocytes which, as stated earlier, are immunologically specific with receptors for the antigens. These reactions occur 12–48 hours after the exposure to the antigen, hence are termed delayed hypersensitivity reactions. Examples are contact dermatitis or the skin test used in suspected cases of tuberculosis.

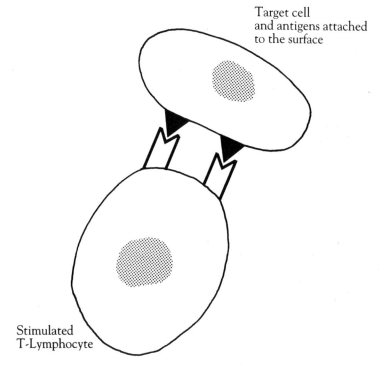

Target cell
and antigens attached
to the surface

Stimulated
T-Lymphocyte

Figure 3.6   Type 4 Reaction

Chapter 4

The Genetic and Environmental Factors in Allergy

There are some definite genetic markers which determine whether a particular infant or child will develop an allergic disorder. These genetic factors are complex and are at present poorly understood. Whatever their nature, the environmental influences are also of paramount importance.

Table 4.1   The risks of developing allergy

	Frequency (%) in child
Both parents having same allergy	70
Both parents having different allergies	45
One parent allergic	20
Both parents non-allergic	10

Identical twins are much more likely to develop asthma or nasal allergies than if they are fraternal twins only. If both parents have, or have had, some allergic disorders the chances that their baby or infant will develop allergy are extremely high — in the order of 40 to 50 per cent. The risks are halved when one parent only is, or has been, affected by an allergic disorder and the risks gradually diminish significantly if family history of allergies is completely absent. Despite the innate predisposition to develop allergy, it is the environment of the family and the child that will influence this susceptibility to allergy. For instance, the baby born during early springtime is much more likely to develop pollen allergy than if s/he were born in the autumn or winter months. Also, babies who are artificially fed (i.e. on cow's milk) develop virus infections of the respiratory tract during the first year of life much more commonly than babies who are completely breast fed. These virus infections have a tendency to cause undue and persistent irritation of the infant's respiratory passages for many months. Some of these infants progress to develop asthma. Similar irritation of the respiratory system is caused by cigarette smoke within the household. Conversely, a baby that is breast fed exclusively for the first few months of life has a good chance of escaping the nastiness of eczema even if both the parents have suffered from some allergies themselves. More recently it has been shown in a group of infants that avoidance of some environmental allergens, such as house dust and animals, and following a modified infant's diet resulted in fewer developing persistent and troublesome eczema during the first two years of life.

Adverse weather conditions, such as frequent changes in air temperature and humidity, pollution of the atmosphere, dampness of living rooms, etc. — all these factors can influence directly the development of allergic disorders. In addition, and practically as important, these factors can be responsible for many exacerbations of already established allergies.

In summary, your baby is more likely to develop allergy if:
- you as a parent have some form of allergy
- your parents have had some well-known allergies
- your baby is born during early spring
- you do not, or did not, breast feed your baby
- you live in a damp house
- you or others smoke cigarettes in the house
- you keep pet animals
- the baby's blood IgE level is very high

Conversely, your baby is less likely to develop allergy if:
- you as a parent have or have had no known allergies
- your parents have or have had no established allergies
- your baby is born during the autumn months
- you breast feed your baby for a few months
- your baby has avoided contact with pet animals for the first few months of life
- the baby's blood IgE level is fairly low
- you have been careful in introducing weaning foods

Chapter 5

How Common are Allergies in Children?

Up to 20 per cent of all children become affected by one of the major allergic disorders before they reach adolescence.

FOOD ALLERGY

The exact incidence remains unknown. During the first year of life about 2 per cent of all newborn babies develop allergy to cow's milk. The baby may develop nasal snuffles, eczema, and breathing problems such as rapid respirations or wheeze. Most of the cow's milk allergies are of the acute or immediate type, i.e. they occur very soon after the drinking of the milk. In some babies, however, delayed types of reaction may also be produced, i.e. recurrent symptoms not readily ascribed to cow's milk, such as abdominal colic, occasional vomiting and/or diarrhoea, wheezy chest. These signs and symptoms usually clear up or considerably improve between feeds. The reason why babies become allergic to cow's milk is related to the immaturity of the various immunological processes in the baby's gastrointestinal tract so that the baby can be fairly easily sensitized to the foreign proteins. As the infant grows older and the immune processes of the gut mature, many food allergies become less of a problem. Hence the common finding that food allergies tend to improve spontaneously with age. However, some food allergies can persist inexplicably for many years and even for a lifetime.

John, aged 11 years, had always been a healthy boy who rather enjoyed the occasional meal of fish and chips — until one day. As soon as he placed a morsel of fish in his mouth, he noticed a burning and tingling sensation in his throat and

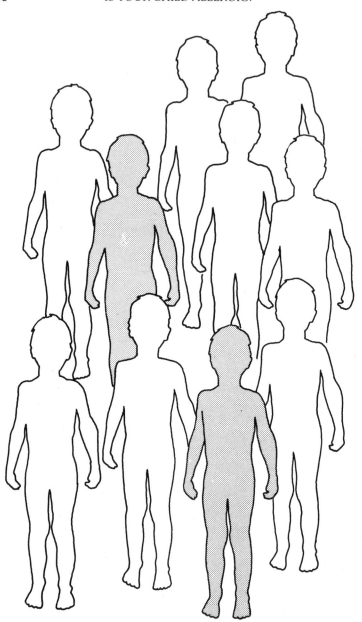

Figure 5.1   Remember: Your child is not alone

Your child and his allergy have plenty of company. The number of substances to which any one of us can develop allergies is increasing year by year — new fabrics, cosmetics, preservatives, pesticides, plastics, air pollutants — are just a few offenders.

his lips began to swell. He thought that he had burned himself with the chips, so he rested a while and a little later he tried again. This time he started to feel really ill — his face started to swell rapidly and he felt like scratching it all over. Soon a burning red rash appeared on his face. His parents became alarmed by his grotesque appearance and initially felt he must have been stung by a bee. They rushed him to hospital. By the time he was being examined, everyone could hear him wheeze and the red rash had spread to other parts of his body. He responded quickly to emergency treatment. Detailed tests showed that John had become allergic to a type of flat fish (flounder) which he had had on two or three previous occasions only, but he could eat other unrelated types of fish or shellfish. Nonetheless he was advised to avoid in future all types of fish and fish products.

Six years later he inadvertently took a bite of a salmon paste sandwich. Within minutes acute symptoms appeared requiring urgent treatment. Further enquiries showed that the 'salmon' was a mixture of fish! At the age of 22 he made a similar mistake!

Comment: About 70 per cent of children become allergic to fish of the same species, e.g. bony fish. The other 30 per cent can tolerate other species of fish. The case history illustrates dramatically that fish allergy can persist and cause severe symptoms for many years — in John's case for 11 years already.

ALLERGIC SKIN CONDITIONS

In general, 5-10 per cent of infants and children develop skin allergies before reaching adolescence.

There are two broad groups of allergic skin conditions:
1. Eczema (atopic dermatitis or 'itch that rashes') and allergies produced by a direct contact with an allergen (contact dermatitis).
2. Hives (urticaria, from the Latin 'urtica' — nettle) and acute swelling of the body tissues (angioedema).

Between 3 and 5 per cent of children under 5 years of age develop eczema and of these 70 per cent do so before their second birthday. Eczema almost completely clears in 60-70 per cent of children by the age of 5 years. If eczema persists over the age of 5 or 6 years it is likely to continue causing problems for many years to come. The true incidence of contact dermatitis in children is not fully known — perhaps between 2 and 4 per cent.

Hives (nettle type rashes) occur in 2-3 per cent of children. Between 10-20 per cent of the population develop the condition sometime during their lives. Acute swelling of tissues may be associated with hives and occurs in 1 to 2 per cent of children.

ASTHMA

About 10 per cent of children develop asthma. The majority of children acquire it before the age of 6-8 years. Boys are affected twice as often as girls, but the order becomes reversed by late adolescence and early adulthood. There is a tendency towards spontaneous improvement of asthma with age so that by late teens, about 30-50 per cent of individuals become free of symptoms of asthma — some for ever, some for many years, some only for a few months or years. Some adolescents develop other types of allergies during this time in their life. For these reasons, I never tell parents and older children that they will 'outgrow their asthma'—they are more likely to outgrow their doctors first! About 25-30 children die each year from the effects of asthma in England and Wales.

NASAL ALLERGIES

These occur in 5-10 per cent of children under 15 years of age. Seasonal allergies (hay fever) are at least two or three times more common than non-seasonal, i.e. perennial allergies. In grass pollen allergy there is a tendency for spontaneous and long-term remissions with each season. The majority of children lose their hay fever symptoms after five to eight seasons. Thirty to forty per cent of children with perennial rhinitis develop symptoms before their tenth birthday and the symptoms tend to persist for more years than in seasonal rhinitis. Boys and girls are equally affected. Also, the child with recurrent or chronic nasal allergies may develop inflammation of the sinuses, a persistent cough, often at night, nasal discharge of mucus, sore throat, or glue ear.

DRUG ALLERGIES

Drug reactions may occur because of true allergy, toxicity or idiosyncrasy. The true incidence of drug reactions in children is unknown. Minor reactions are fairly common — about 5-10 per cent. Some children with asthma become allergic to aspirin and products containing aspirin. The symptoms of drug allergy may vary from a sudden collapse of the child to transient skin rashes of various forms, persistent feverish episodes or joint swellings.

INSECT ALLERGY

Allergic reactions to insect bites or stings are very common in children but often remain unrecognized unless they are associated with generalized symptoms and signs such as a skin rash and swelling of tissues, breathing difficulties or acute collapse of the child. The most serious reactions are caused by bee and wasp stings. These account for three to five fatalities each year in the United Kingdom and about forty deaths a year in the United States. The most common insect bites are caused by fleas which are blood sucking insects living on animals and man. They are very active during the summer months and cause an itch and a spotty reddish rash which when carefully inspected with a magnifying glass will have a tiny puncture in the centre which is visibly swollen.

ARE ALLERGIES EVER OUTGROWN?

Some parents believe mistakenly that if they do nothing about their children's allergies these 'will go away'. This apparent neglect results in the child continuing to have various allergy problems from infancy to childhood. Infant colic may be replaced later on by food allergy, eczema may be followed by asthma which may become spasmodic initially to be followed later on by almost continual respiratory disease leading to frequent school absences and emotional problems. The so-called 'colds' may continue throughout every season of the year, or lead to attacks of asthma at certain times of the year. Thus it is essential to identify children's allergies early in life so that adequate treatment can be instituted which may result in allowing the child to enjoy as normal a life as his non-allergic companions.

HOW CAN ALLERGIC DISORDERS BE PREVENTED IN CHILDREN?

1. Breast feed your baby exclusively. If you suffer, or have suffered, from chronic allergies yourself, or you have a very strong family history of allergies, and especially if your previous baby developed an allergic disorder, you may wish to consider putting yourself on an exclusive diet so as to avoid milk and its products, wheat, eggs, nuts and so on. Occasionally such strict measures are helpful. It is absolutely essential to consult an experienced doctor or dietitian if you are proposing to try such a regimen, as otherwise you are likely to develop malnutrition and subsequently your baby will thrive poorly. Do not accept reckless recommendations or advice, however well-meaning, from unprofessional individuals. During the last few years I have seen some tragic cases.

> Mrs A. has had asthma all her life and her first son Bruce developed severe eczema during the first year of life and then at about 3 years of age, asthma. Bruce required frequent medical attention but managed to grow relatively satisfactorily. When Mrs A. became pregnant again she decided to start herself on a special diet during the last month of her pregnancy. She read about the diet and the wonders it achieved in a magazine. So when Frank was born she started to breast feed him completely. At the age of 3 months Frank started to develop patches of eczema — first on his face and scalp and then on other parts of the body. He started to cry incessantly and become difficult to console. Most of the time he appeared restless and on the go. Mrs. A consulted a herbalist and some remedies were tried but without success. One day she had a visit from the health visitor who was shocked to find both mother and baby thin and the mother herself on the verge of desperation. The baby's weight was within the 'Belsen' range. Both the mother and baby were admitted to hospital for tests which

showed that the baby's milk intake was grossly inadequate, not only because of the mother's anxieties but also because of Frank's generalized restlessness due to the severe discomfort and itching which he developed from the infected eczema.

Comment: This is one of a number of typical problems that occur when parents, for one reason or another, do not seek professional advice. These mothers and their babies need a great deal of sympathy and understanding from everyone, but it is important not to do harm by 'off the cuff' advice. Many babies breast fed exclusively do well but some, for reasons which remain at present unclear, do not — all the more reason then to be guided by an experienced dietitian and adviser.

2. If there is a history of food allergy alone in the family, exclude milk and its products, wheat and eggs from the baby's diet during the first year of life. Ensure that the baby's diet is otherwise nutritionally adequate, and that the diet contains all the vitamins essential for growth. Avoid additives and preservatives throughout the first 18 months of life.

After the first year of life, add new foods to the infant's diet one by one — every four or five days — and note any untoward effects. If the infant develops diarrhoea because of a virus or bacterial infection, reduce or stop the intake of these common protein-containing foods because the baby's gastrointestinal tract at that time becomes very inflamed and thus allows the various offending protein molecules to be absorbed into the bloodstream.

3. Avoid unnecessary medications. If you do use them — read the instructions carefully to find what they contain and why they should be used.

4. Institute house dust mite avoidance measures (p. 87). Some children with eczema get worse when exposed to the house dust mite.

5. Avoid cigarette smoking throughout pregnancy and in the household once the baby is born.
Smoking by pregnant women:
- affects the baby's growth in the womb. The baby is smaller all round — head size, chest, and limbs, and it is lighter than a baby born to a mother who does not smoke
- the more cigarettes, the lighter the baby

- constitutes a risk factor for the Sudden Infant Death Syndrome (cot death)

Smoke is an irritant to the baby's nasal and breathing passages and predisposes him to develop chest infections.

Chapter 6

Food Allergy

The development of effective measures of preventing foods from being infected or contaminated by microbes, i.e. refrigeration, and the addition of preservatives, etc. has resulted, in most industrialized societies, in a significant reduction of adverse reactions to foods associated with infections. Sporadic instances of food poisoning still occur when we fail to follow these preventive measures diligently. However, the modern man has gradually introduced a large variety of substances into the daily foodstuffs, albeit for reasons which at times are not readily apparent. Thus, the child may become truly allergic to some of these added ingredients because of repeated exposure or because of the chemical or complex structure of the ingredients which he may not be able to tolerate.

It follows, therefore, that adverse food reaction may be:

Truly allergic
— acute and sudden following exposure to the offending food. (Immediate Allergic Reaction).
— delayed. Occurring hours or even days after food ingestion.

Non-allergic (food intolerance)
— easily identifiable because the child may be lacking an enzyme to digest a particular food, e.g. some sugars, or the substance contains powerful pharmacological substances, e.g. strawberries contain histamine and may be responsible for abdominal pains and bouts of diarrhoea.
— 'proven' on circumstantial evidence because of lack of specific and conclusive tests. For instance, just because the child's headaches improve temporarily when the diet is altered

by the removal of some suspected food substances does not prove intolerance—it may be a sheer coincidence or a psychologically motivated phenomenon.

Adverse food reactions are summarized in Table 6.1.

Table 6.1   Adverse reactions to foods

Food allergy (IgE mediated)	Food intolerance (non-immunologically caused)
Toxicity	Idiosyncrasy
Deficient Enzyme	
Immediate reactions	Delayed reactions

Acute food allergy symptoms are produced as a result of immunological reactions which are fairly well understood. The delayed allergic food reactions remain to be worked out fully and the knowledge of the immunological mechanisms involved is poorly understood. The understanding of the mechanisms of adverse reactions to foods caused by intolerance is either straightforward or totally unknown—hence the reason for the genuine problems of diagnosis and management.

SYMPTOMS OF FOOD ALLERGY

Clara, aged 4 months, was a perfectly normal baby. She was the first child of parents whose father had a history of asthma as a child. The mother had a tendency to occasional episodes of headaches which she interpreted as migraine because they responded to aspirin or rest. It was about this time that Clara's father became rather depressed because of rumours that he might lose his office job. Clara's mother sensed that her husband was unhappy, despite the fact that he did not discuss the matter with her, and she quickly realized that she was being affected as well. Clara, who was fully breast fed, started to cry two or three hours after feeds, became restless and appeared to develop loose motions. A discussion with the doctor and the practice nurse revealed that Clara was not gaining weight adequately because 'Mum's milk was drying up'. All appeared well for a few weeks, after which Clara started to develop nasal snuffles which were initially thought to be 'colds', wheezy chests, and an unpleasant rash on her face, body and legs. Hospital tests confirmed that Clara was allergic to some of the proteins of cow's milk, and her symptoms and signs cleared up completely on a modified diet. At the age of 19 months she was able to tolerate cow's milk and its products in the foods which the mother gave her from time to time.

Comment: Clara's history demonstrates the variety of signs and symptoms which may be produced by adverse food reactions. Some children may not give such clear-cut histories. They may complain of aches and pains, indigestion, abdominal pains, headaches, tiredness and so on. Although these symptoms may suggest an allergic explanation, it is essential for parents to remember that there are other equally important treatable medical conditions which must be taken into consideration when a differential diagnosis is made.

The most common foods responsible for reactions are:
cow's milk
eggs (as a rule egg white only)
cheese
chocolate
wheat
fish and shellfish
nuts (and peanut butter)
vegetables — (peas)
fruits (especially tomatoes, strawberries, pineapple and citrus)
mushrooms
yeast
spices and seasonings
food additives
drugs — which may be inadvertently found in foods

Foods that rarely cause allergies:
polished rice
lamb meat
lettuce
The multiple variety of symptoms and signs attributed to adverse food reactions are summarized in Table 6.2.

Table 6.2   Symptoms and signs which suggest food allergy

1. Mouth
   Ulcers
   Swelling of the tongue
   Patchy areas of excessive redness

2. Stomach and intestines
   Spasm of the muscle between the stomach and small
      intestine, causing recurrent vomiting
   Recurrent colicky pains
   Diarrhoea and/or vomiting
   Passage of blood in stools
   Indigestion and flatulence
   Recurrent passage of blood and/or mucus with motions

3. Skin
   Hives and swelling of tissues
   Eczema

4. Respiratory system
   Nasal problems
   Ear problems (glue ear)
   Asthma

5. Blood
   Anaemia

6. Nervous system
   Migraine
   Hyperactivity
   Tension-fatigue

7. Kidneys
   Bed-wetting
   Passage of protein and/or blood in the urine

8. Other (some controversial)
   Cot death or sudden death
   Recurrent arthritis

WHAT TO DO IF YOU THINK YOUR CHILD MIGHT BE FOOD SENSITIVE

Get a pencil and paper and write down the symptoms your baby or child has had for as long as you can remember. If you have already been to your doctor and were given some treatment, make sure you know exactly what the treatment was and what benefits, if any, were produced.

Cast your mind back to your childhood. Did you have any recurrent illnesses which were either diagnozed as allergies, e.g. asthma, eczema, hay fever, or did you as it were 'grow out of recurrent bouts of coughing', the nature of which has remained a mystery? Check on your family histories. Obtain similar information from the father (or vice versa) and his family. Then turn to your other children — have they or have they had recurrent problems that might suggest adverse food effects?

Check your child's diet details. If you have difficulty in remembering all that he eats, the best and easiest way is to carry on normally and keep a written record of what is being eaten. The record should include everything — school dinners, drinks between meals, etc. If you are not sure of the accuracy — say so. Keep a record for at least 14 days. The information that you obtain may form a sound basis for diagnosis and effective treatment.

Once you have obtained a history and a record of food eaten, seek medical advice. Tell your doctor of the child's symptoms, explain positive family history and show him the food records that you have kept.

The doctor cannot dismiss your fears or anxieties of suspected food allergy or intolerance without a thorough examination, full face explanations of how the symptoms arose or otherwise by performing further laboratory tests if needed. At times a referral to an expert may be required to prove or disprove your suspicions.

It is most important to seek experienced professional medical advice since the prescription of diets and dubious forms of treatments to children, which are based on flimsy evidence, can at best be useless and at times most dangerous.

Sean, aged 4 years 9 months, had just started at his local school. He had a tendency to asthma and eczema and was described by his parents as being a 'bit of a worrier'. Soon after starting school he developed recurrent headaches—from time to time, sometimes in the morning, sometimes on coming home from school. On occasions he felt tired and moody. To add to parental worry, his eczema started to play up and his coughing became more frequent during the night. Sean's teachers confirmed the mother's suspicions that 'it all has to do with starting school, after all many children are like that' — hence she took no further action until one day when his eczema got worse. Instead of taking him to her regular doctor she consulted an untrained individual who offered (without explanation) a number of remedies. A few days later Sean refused to wake up in the morning — he appeared drowsy and confused. A visiting doctor advised urgent hospital admission. Detailed investigations revealed a brain tumour which thankfully was of a low degree of malignancy so that it could be completely removed. Sean recovered fully from his brain tumour. He continued to have occasional episodes of asthma and eczema until 12 years of age when his asthma ceased to be a problem and he was left with the odd patch of eczema over his elbows and knees.

Comment: Jumping to conclusions without a thorough assessment is a practice we can all do without.

WHAT OTHER TESTS ARE NEEDED TO CONFIRM ALLERGY OR FOOD INTOLERANCE?

Skin prick tests can be done for particular food allergens. Unfortunately these tests are often unhelpful and confusion may arise when a test may become positive to a food which the child can eat without any problems. The one great value of this test is in children who are said to be allergic to chicken eggs. A confirmatory skin test will forewarn the parents and the doctors that strict precautions should be taken when any vaccines or immunizations are given to the child as severe and general reactions can occur. The doctor can dilute the vaccine, or if necessary, use a vaccine cultured on duck eggs or other species.

The practice of injecting food extracts under the skin or placing them under the child's tongue gives unreliable and non-specific responses and may be alarming. Similarly, an analysis of samples of hair for food allergens is of no practical value at all.

A blood sample can be taken from the child and tested for specific IgE antibodies to particular foods. The best results are obtained in children with allergic hives. The tests are called radioallergosorbent test (or RAST) and paper immunosorbent test (or PRIST).

Where the clinical history and examination indicates, tests of the gastrointestinal function may be required. The baby's or infant's stools can be examined for sugars, fats, bacteria, blood, etc. At times a tiny sample of the small intestine can be taken and examined for structure, signs of inflammation, damage and the presence or absence of digestive enzymes. This simple procedure is usually carried out without the need of a hospital admission, and consists of passing a plastic tube to which a capsule is attached through the mouth to the stomach and then just passing it to the small intestine. The modern and sophisticated X-ray facilities allow the capsule to be observed carefully and a sample of the superficial lining of the intestine (biopsy) is obtained for examination. The procedure does not cause any pain to the child — it does irritate the throat a little as the tube is passed to the stomach. However, the information obtained from the biopsy is often diagnostic — as in the intolerance to gluten which is present in wheat or rye flour (also called coeliac disease) or in an infant allergic to cow's milk proteins, or intolerant to the sugars present in the milk.

FOOD ELIMINATION AND PROVOCATION TESTING

These procedures can be helpful in unravelling delayed food allergies. Provocation testing, i.e. challenging the child with a suspected offending food can be very dangerous in situations where the child has experienced acute or immediate reactions. You should ensure that the preliminary tests as outlined above have been performed and were normal. The success rate of using food challenges for the diagnosis of delayed allergy is about 40 to 50 per cent. A positive diagnosis is suspected when the symptoms completely disappear as the offending food is withdrawn from the child's diet; they reappear within 48 hours or so if the food is re-introduced, and most importantly, the signs and symptoms are always similar in nature. Some doctors prefer to repeat two or three challenges and withdrawals.

However, in children who have a variety of frequent and recurrent symptoms of uncertain causation, it is not possible to carry out a worthwhile challenge test — a 'suspected' food-free period is needed. This is obtained by placing the child on a diet containing food of low-allergenicity for 14-21 days. If symptoms disappear, the suspicions of allergy or intolerance are strengthened. Subsequently, batches of new foods are introduced to the diet depending whether any new symptoms develop or not. As can be appreciated, these procedures are fairly exacting, time-consuming and require the services of a trained children's dietitian and other experts. An example of low-allergen exclusion diet is shown in Table 6.3.

Table 6.3   Low allergen exclusion diet

Allowed only   (no additives, preservatives)
                        polished rice
                        gluten-free bread
                        olive oil
                        cooked chicken
                        honey
                        fresh fruit (except apples, citrus)
                        vegetables (except peas)
                        barley and cane sugar
                        salt
                        water (pure)

                        Tomor Margarine (free of butter)
                        (Kosher)

A number of modifications of low-allergen diet have been described. Some authorities use artificial diets containing amino acids, glucose and vitamins.

In certain situations, and easily used as a home procedure, is the employment of the so-called double-blind provocation test. The parents are given a series of numbered capsules containing various amounts of dried foods and substances, e.g. eggs, wheat, additives, etc. Each capsule is taken in the morning and any symptoms are observed for two to four hours and recorded by the parents throughout the next 20 hours. With each completed series, and provided no symptoms appear, the dosage of a particular substance is increased and the cycle repeated. Such an approach will detect the majority of children allergic or intolerant to foods. But there are some exceptions — for instance, some children with migraine attacks require to be on a food exclusion diet for five to eight weeks before they lose their symptoms and at other times sensitivity to some foods may be worse in one week and less so in another — hence interpretations of the tests can be extremely difficult and require a great deal of expertise.

SOME SPECIFIC FOOD ALLERGY OR INTOLERANCE PROBLEMS

Cow's milk allergy

Occurs in about 1 per cent of all babies. Boys are affected twice as commonly as girls. If one baby in a family has cow's milk allergy, the chances of a similar problem in a brother or sister are about 50 per cent. The cow's milk contains at least 50 allergic proteins of which only a few have been fully studied. Sensitivity to a beta-lactoglobulin is the most frequently encountered problem.

The baby is usually under 1 year of age and has frequent symptoms such as vomiting, diarrhoea, skin rashes or eczema, cough and/or wheeze, poor weight gain, excessive crying, listlessness, abdominal colic, etc. In short, a number of target organs have been involved — the skin, the gastrointestinal tract and the lungs. Some babies may have many symptoms, others only one or two, such as wheeze and snuffles.

At least 90 per cent of babies fully recover by 18-24 months of age — even if not treated or poorly managed. However, proper dietary treatment allows the baby to recover much faster. If the recovery is delayed beyond 2 years of age it is essential to consult your doctor because some of these infants go on to develop gluten sensitivity (coeliac disease).

Some babies who are fully breast fed may develop allergy symptoms because certain food ingredients in the mother's diet, such as cow's milk proteins, egg proteins or drugs or even some substances in beverages if taken to excess may be passed on to the baby during feeds. It is worth remembering also that the nicotine from cigarettes passes into the breast milk and can cause diarrhoea and vomiting and an acceleration of the baby's heart beat.

If any mother suspects that her baby may have allergy to cow's milk she should:

a. Discuss the matter fully with the baby's doctor.
b. Obtain as convincing proof of allergy as possible.
c. Seek to discuss the diet with a qualified dietitian.
d. Ensure a regular supervision of the baby's progress.
e. Check carefully the correct procedure when cow's milk is eventually re-introduced after many months abstinence. This is most important because some babies develop a violent and life-threatening reaction — hence emergency facilities should always be available.

The cavalier practice of replacing one milk product with another in the hope that 'it will do the job' often results in the deterioration of the baby's well-being and causes misery to the parents.

> *Anna, aged 4 months, had never been a happy baby — she was described as a windy baby who cried a great deal as if in pain, slept poorly, occasionally vomited after and between feeds, and was perpetually snuffly. 'She gets one cold after another,' her mother said. Anna's mother tried initially to feed her herself but gave up after nine days because the baby remained unsettled. She tried one respected cow's milk formula for two weeks but Anna appeared to be 'a little worse' although she did gain some weight. Someone advised a change of milk. So she tried again, but Anna was no better after a week. A trial of goat's milk appeared initially to 'have done the job'. Three weeks later she was as bad as on the first milk product. Her symptoms were now more frequent —her breathing had become quite noisy and was a somewhat frightening experience at night so that Anna's cot was brought back from her room to the parent's bedroom. Soon Dad was getting agitated by disturbed nights, adding further to Mum's anxiety state. A desperate visit to a doctor for advice resulted in a diagnosis of throat infection and a prescription for an antibiotic. Two days later Anna developed profuse diarrhoea and was sent to the local hospital. While all her fluids and nourishment were being given through a vein her symptoms of snuffles, vomiting, diarrhoea and disturbed breathing improved rapidly. As soon as she was home again her symptoms returned. The health visitor suggested a special milk substitute made from soya protein. About one month later, at a time when Anna's parents were gloating at her excellent health, the*

symptoms returned yet again, and this time with a vengeance requiring emergency hospital care.

Comment: Tests showed that Anna did have cow's milk protein allergy and was also allergic to the soya milk. Such special milks are at times allergic themselves and importantly they may interfere in producing a satisfactory antibody response in the blood when the baby is immunized, e.g. against polio, diphtheria, tetanus and whooping cough. About one in ten babies allergic to cow's milk will also develop allergy to the soya protein. Some babies allergic to cow's milk proteins can respond to goat's milk. The claims for goat's milk's usefulness are often based on folklore. Indeed, some of the proteins both in cow's milk and goat's milk are very similar in their immunological composition — e.g. when given to guinea pigs the adverse reactions are indistinguishable. However, the fatty acids in goat's milk are well digested by human babies. The milk contains more fat than either the human or the cow's milk but, in total, it provides the same energy value as human milk.

Abdominal colic (Also called infant colic, three months or evening colic. Derived from the word 'colon', i.e. large intestine, 'colicky' pains come most commonly from the small intestine!)

This involves recurrent bouts of abdominal pain, of varying intensity but short duration, during which the baby may become extremely distressed — crying uncontrollably, almost impossible to pacify, poorly responsive to comforting gestures. The pains occur because of the distension or stretching of the gastrointestinal tract. Possibly the most common cause is hunger of the underfed baby who swallows excessive amounts of air. But there are many other explanations, and allergy to cow's milk is occasionally the cause irrespective of whether the baby is breast or bottle fed. Often there is a history of allergies in the other members of the family.

A mother who breast feeds may pass the foreign cow's milk proteins to her baby in the milk. Thus removal of cow's milk and its products from the mother's diet can be curative.

A baby fed with a cow's milk formula responds very well to special cow's milk substitutes, e.g. hydrolyzed protein milk containing sugars such as glucose or sucrose for easier digestion.

It was a Sunday evening in November when Caroline, aged 2 months, disturbed suddenly the evening's TV proceedings. She was put to the breast as usual, fed well, and appeared contented as she lay in her cot. A few minutes later she became acutely agitated — her face became intensely red, her tummy appeared to swell up and she started to perform rapid movements with her legs. These events were matched by bouts of distressed and loud cries. She was difficult to console and when she unexpectedly vomited a little amount of milk her mother phoned for the doctor. The parents were told Caroline had a colic, were given a medicine to help her and asked to report if she did not improve. Unfortunately she did not. Her symptoms continued on and off day after day despite changes in drug management. In desperation the mother consulted a chemist, and then a practitioner of homoeopathy — but it was all to no avail. A home consultation with a specialist was arranged. Although definitive evidence of cow's milk protein allergy could not be immediately proven, the mother was put on a diet excluding cow's milk and its products, eggs and additives. Within 48 hours Caroline's symptoms ceased. Subsequent results of the baby's blood tests confirmed high levels of IgE.

Comment: The majority of babies with colicky abdominal pains improve with simple measures and sound advice. Some may have other reasons — cow's milk allergy is one of them. When in doubt discuss the matter with your doctor as it is essential to examine the baby during a bout in order to exclude all the serious surgical abdominal conditions.

In another patient, the baby's problems ceased when the mother took sodium cromoglycate (see p. 117) before each feed. It would probably have been better to give the drug to the baby before feeds.

Irritable Bowel Syndrome (Toddler's diarrhoea, also non-specific diarrhoea).

Many infants, otherwise healthy and growing satisfactorily, have recurrent bouts of diarrhoea, often for days, or even weeks, and which are characterized by the passage of frequent and unformed stools containing vegetable and fruit fibre such as carrots, peas, sweet corn, and oranges, etc. True allergy is most uncommon.

The nature of this condition is not fully known and since the symptoms simulate other chronic bowel disorders, some infants undergo many tests which are helpful in that they exclude these disorders but they do not help in shedding further light on the exact causation of the syndrome. There are various beneficial approaches to the management of this condition. A thorough examination of the child and assessment of progress are needed rather than a trial of diverse remedies of dubious practical value.

Coeliac disease (from Greek 'Koilia' meaning belly).

The relationship of this condition to allergy remains to be worked out. There exist definite genetic factors. For instance, about 10 per cent of close relatives may have similar problems. Girls and boys are equally affected and by their third birthday at least 50 per cent develop clinical symptoms. The condition arises because of a specific intolerance to a gluten fraction which is a protein found particularly in wheat, rye and oat flour. In these genetically susceptible infants and young children gluten is toxic to the fine lining of the digestive tract and causes offensive diarrhoea containing lots of fat and protein. The infant either does not gain weight or loses it gradually. The clinical picture depends on the severity and the duration of symptoms. A jejunal biopsy (p. 45) is diagnostic and the response to a gluten free diet is excellent. The diet needs to be continued throughout life or until such time when a definitive breakthrough in the understanding of the condition finally occurs.

Allergic proctitis

Some infants and children develop intense irritation, discomfort and discharge of mucus from the last few centimetres of the back passage, i.e. rectum. Detailed tests often reveal IgE cells in the lining of the gut. Some workers believe the condition is due to allergens in the baby's stools. The disorder responds favourably to an anti-allergic management.

Allergic Tension-Fatigue Syndrome

During the last 30 years a number of reports have appeared in the medical literature suggesting that some infants and children develop a specific condition characterized by alternating periods of tension and excessive fatigue and that these and other symptoms (see Table 6.4) are due to a delayed-onset food allergy, e.g. due to wheat, eggs, cola drinks, etc. and that the elimination of some of these particular foods leads to a considerable improvement, the return of well-being and disappearance of the symptoms.

Since definitive diagnostic tests are not available, a controversy exists among many specialists whether this plethora of symptoms is due to a true allergy, or a non-allergic reaction to some foods, or are part and parcel of the normal growing up of young children. There is no doubt that a number of specific agents in food can cause similar symptoms. For instance, recurrent headaches, sleep problems and tummy pains can be caused by substances present in bananas, pineapples, tomatoes and cheese, tea, coffee, chocolates, cola drinks, liquorice, etc. Here the identity of the particular and naturally occurring pharmacological agent is usually fairly obvious when a detailed history is taken. Some children have also been described who developed exacerbations of symptoms during the spring and summer months only and children who were shown to be allergic to various inhalants such as the house dust mite, house dust, feathers, mould spores and animal dander.

The issue has been confused further by the observations that some of these children, in addition to being tense and fatigued, have become extremely overactive (hyperactive).

I have observed a number of children who have manifested some features of odd behaviour, sleep disturbance and restlessness but all of them had asthma and/or eczema and nasal allergies. In most situations the behaviour problems improved as the other conditions were properly assessed, investigated and treated effectively. However, there is no doubt that some children with asthma, for instance, do develop non-respiratory symptoms before attacks of asthma. Possibly these symptoms are due to the release of pharmacological substances which act on other target organs of the body.

Jane, aged 8 years 2 months, had had asthma and eczema for most of her life. She had had various treatments which undoubtedly helped her from time to time. On occasions, and for no obvious reasons, she would deteriorate rapidly — the cycle of events was most characteristic. First her eczema would get worse for a day or two and then asthma would start. It was most unusual for Jane to develop asthma either first or asthma alone. It became apparent that the control of eczema prevented attacks of asthma but not the other way round. Further revelations followed. Jane's mother observed that before the eczema rash appeared, Jane would become very restless at night ('she has restless legs') and in the morning she would develop an intense desire to scratch her shoulders and arms, she would become unruly, aggressive and 'rather nasty'. Although it was difficult to prove conclusively whether Jane was allergic to some foods and other agents, the levels of histamine in her blood during one episode were markedly elevated, suggesting that some form of allergy played a part in the causation of her exacerbations of eczema and asthma. Although drugs and other medications controlled the acute symptoms effectively, they did not prevent recurrences. A controlled diet avoiding milk, egg, corn, wheat, refined sugars, additives and preservatives was associated with episodes of prolonged improvement of symptoms but inexplicably occasional relapses continued to occur up to the age of 14 years when exacerbations of eczema would not be followed by attacks of asthma despite the fact that the respiratory function tests showed that Jane's breathing tubes could still respond adversely to an allergen challenge.

Comment: The history demonstrates that many organs can be affected during an 'allergic' attack. I suppose we concentrate most on the organ causing the most severe symptoms and tend to forget others. Secondly, it is not uncommon for some children to develop prodromal (from Latin 'dromos' meaning forerunner) symptoms before an attack of asthma, e.g. scratching of the head, neck, etc. Thirdly, Jane did display some features of tension-fatigue but I was never convinced that these symptoms occurred separately and formed an entity of their own.

The hyperactive child

Michael had always been an active infant. His mother noticed the change when he reached his second birthday. Despite full days of activity he seemed to carry on. His sister Emma, two years older, usually flopped to sleep straight away. Michael did not. Nothing appeared to make him happy. His mother became tired and weary and made frequent visits to the doctor for sedatives and other pacifying

Table 6.4   Some common Tension-Fatigue symptoms

Tension
>   Overactive
>   Clumsy
>   Cannot relax
>   Cannot concentrate
>   Irritable
>   Oversensitive
>   Poor sleeper

Fatigue
>   Sluggish
>   Tired

Other symptoms which may be present
>   General lassitude
>   Headaches
>   Aches and pains
>   Bed-wetting
>   Mood changes
>   Behaviour problems
>   Persistent nasal congestion

medicines in order to keep him calm. Nothing seemed to help. She hoped he would improve as he grew older, and resigned herself to the role of supporting him throughout the day and to many sleepless nights. But Michael's boisterous activities continued to increase — he appeared as if driven by some secret engine — always on the go, always climbing up and down chairs or running purposelessly about. Games appeared to excite him a great deal and he found it difficult to calm down afterwards. The story-time and bedtime became an ordeal for everyone as Michael, initially attentive, would become fidgety and disruptive. A trusted baby-sitter declined to look after him as he wore her out and she was afraid she might hit him in desperation. Although he eventually would manage to get off to sleep, the hours of the night were full of restless groans and moans and fidgetiness. At times sedatives were most helpful, at other times they were ineffective.

Another few months and Michael would have to go to school. This fearful prospect prompted the parents to seek further medical advice. Extensive tests revealed that Michael was of normal intelligence, a rather immature boy who had high serum IgE levels despite the fact that he did not show any obvious allergies like asthma or skin problems. He was found to be intolerant to tartrazine, a food colourant (E102) when challenged in a blind fashion. An eight week food elimination diet resulted in a significant improvement in Michael's behaviour and sleep pattern. The parents were advised to exclude all food additives on a permanent basis. At the age of 6 years he developed clinical asthma which was controlled easily on established medications — colour-free, of course. He continues otherwise to enjoy relatively normal health.

Comment: Michael's problem was fairly straightforward but it took some time to establish. The problem can be complex and many children do not respond so well. Other means have to be carefully considered and they can be very beneficial.

The word hyperactivity means, literally, too much activity — thus it is a pattern of behaviour displayed by some children. However, some workers changed this descriptive word into a diagnostic label—implying a definitive disorder and hence requiring an appropriate treatment. Other terms have been introduced during the last few years — e.g. the hyperkinetic syndrome, impulse disorder, minimal brain dysfunction, attention-deficit disorder.

Most parents, teachers, psychologists and doctors can tell easily whether a child is overactive, but it can be extremely difficult to prove whether such hyperactivity is a variant of 'normal' child activities because we do not have any normal standards of activity in children and we have not developed any repetitive ways of measuring overactive or impulsive children. Also, the response to various treatments can be difficult to assess objectively. Nonetheless, a number of children do appear to have an 'excess' of complex symptoms of many months' duration which cause tremendous management problems to parents and teachers. It is essential, therefore, to assess each child and family very carefully and then proceed to an appropriate form of treatment.

The condition is best considered as a developmental disorder, i.e. early onset at between two and five years of age, often with a history of abdominal colic, restlessness. The overactivity is frequently first commented upon when the child, often a boy, attends a nursery school, e.g. 's/he cannot sit still', 'poor attention', 'impulsive' or s/he may appear to have learning problems, become unmanageable, or act in a very immature way despite his/her age. Some common and persistent symptoms of the hyperactivity disorder are given in Table 6.5. In general, infants and young children usually have a greater number of symptoms than most older children.

Estimates of hyperactive behaviour among primary school-children vary from one country to another. One would expect to find one hyperactive child in a class of 30 pupils.

Table 6.5   Some common symptoms of the 5-8 year old

1. Hyperactive
   - Always on the go
   - Fidgety most of the time
   - Restless during sleep

2. Inattentive
   - Distracted easily
   - Does not finish things
   - Poor listener
   - Concentrates poorly
   - Games wrecker

3. Impulsive
   - Speaks before thinking
   - Shifts from one thing to another
   - Does not wait his turn during games
   - Disorganized
   - Needs constant supervision

WHAT IS THE PARENT TO DO?

If you think your child may be 'unnaturally' hyperactive, you should consult your doctor and explain your fears. Obtain proper assessment because there can be a number of causes. Food allergy is only one possible explanation. Intolerance to additives, perservatives, refined sugars, are other possible causes. It is entirely wrong, without assessing the child fully, to instigate a severely restricted diet on the off-chance that s/he might improve. I have seen children severely malnourished who had been on restricted diets for no other reason than 's/he suggested I tried it out', or 'have you read about zinc deficiences?'.

FOOD ADDITIVES AND PRESERVATIVES

Some children with asthma or hives (urticaria) can develop clinical exacerbations when given food colouring additives such as tartrazine, sunset yellow, or amaranth, and food preservatives such as benzoic acid derivatives. In addition, many of these children develop generalized symptoms such as weakness, flushing of the skin and face, nasal stuffiness, etc. The amount of additives that a child has to consume to produce symptoms vary. Most children consume about 5-10 mg of tartrazine daily, yet some children can develop symptoms from taking very small amounts, for example after drinking an orange drink which may contain sulphur dioxide as a preservative.

Table 6.6   What are food additives?

Food additive
A substance not normally eaten as food but added to food intentionally for the purpose of preparation, packing, transport, etc., i.e. for technological reasons.

Some common additives are:

a. Preservatives — agents added to foods in order to slow down the growth of bacteria so as to extend their shelf life.

b. Colourings — agents added to foods to make them attractive to the eye.

c. Anti-oxidants — agents added to foods to reduce or prevent acidity so as to avoid early deterioration, e.g. hydroxyanisole butylated, etc.

d. Flavours — agents added to foods to make them appealing to the palate, e.g. monosodium glutamate.

e. Sweeteners — agents added to increase sweetness of foods.

f. Bleach — agents to whiten foods such as bread and flour to make them look attractive.

NOTE ON FOOD LABELLING

The EEC consumer protection programme on food labelling came into force in January 1983. These regulations introduced date marking and a complete list of food ingredients including additives which were either given a chemical name or a serial number — e.g. E102, tartrazine.

The numbers of additives start at E100 and go on to many hundreds. For instance, E925 is chlorine (1984). New numbers are added from time to time. You can obtain a booklet of the full list from:

Ministry of Agriculture
Lion House
Willowburn Trading Estate
Alnwick
Northumberland NE66 2PF (England and Wales)

or

Scottish Home and Health Department
Foods Branch
Room 40
St Andrew's House
Edinburgh EH1 3DE (Scotland)

Also, see *The New E for Additives* by Maurice Hanssen (Thorsons, 1987).

FOOD ADDITIVES AND HYPERACTIVITY

Many years ago, American workers suggested that some hyperactive schoolchildren might be 'sensitive to various artificial food colouring ingredients, flavours and salicylates' (substances derived from salicylic acid possessing a bitter-sweet taste and used in the manufacture of aspirin, some dyes, perfumes and fungicides). The exact way additives affect behaviour has not been defined. The clinical observations of a group of hyperactive children led to the development of a detailed restriction diet — the Feingold (after the doctor), Kaiser-Permanente (after the hospital), or K-P diet.

There is little doubt that some hyperactive children did improve on the diet, but controversy arose when a large group of

Table 6.7   Some food additives known to have caused problems in children

Name	E number	Problem	Source
Acacia (gum arabic)	414	generalized hypersensitivity	cake mix
Aspirin and salicylates		asthma, aspirin sensitivity	lozenges, cakes, jams, ice cream, soft drinks, chewing gum, vinegar
Amaranth (an azo dye)	123	asthma, aspirin sensitivity, hyperactivity	cake mix, soap products, gravy, tinned fruit pies, jelly
A 20 dyes – to give colour to foods. *They include:* azorubine, tartrazine, yellow 2G, sunset yellow, carmoisine, amaranth, ponceau, red 2G, brown FK, chocolate brown, black PN, pigment rubine, quinoline, yellow, erythosine, patent blue, indigo caramine, green S, brilliant blue.	Check respective E numbers	asthma, aspirin sensitivity, hyperactive behaviour	check source carefully
Benzoic acid	210-219	asthma, dermatitis, bowel disturbance, hyperactive behaviour.	jams, syrups, sauces, purées, some yogurt, cheesecakes, soy sauces, orange squashes, coffee essence, some glacé fruits
Caramel	150	hyperactive behaviour	chocolate dessert, biscuits, packet soups, convenience foods, pickled onions, some gravies, pre-packed cakes

Ethyl 4-hydroxy-benzoate	214	asthma, aspirin sensitivity, hyperactive behaviour	dessert sauce, pie fillings, jams, salad cream
Methyl 4-hydroxy-benzoate	218	as above	as above
Monosodium glutamate	621	asthma, skin problems, hyperactive behaviour, high blood pressure	pre-packed snacks, pork pies, sausages, chilli sauces, flavoured noodles
Potassium benzoate	212	asthma, skin problems, hyper-active behaviour	preservative
Potassium hydroxide	525	general sensitivity	cocoa and its products
Potassium nitrate (saltpetre)	252	hyperactive behaviour, skin problems, bowel problems	some meats and sausages, bacon, pressed meats, tinned meats, smoked ham
Propyl benzoate or gallate	216 310	asthma, skin problems, hyperactivity	vegetable oil, breakfast cereals, dessert sauces, freezer drinks, pie fillings, salad cream, soft drinks
Sodium bisulphite	222	asthma	preservative
Tartrazine (see azo dyes)	102	asthma, skin problems, hyperactive behaviour	chewing gum, convenience foods, squashes, tinned peas, salad cream, fizzy drinks, smoked haddock etc.

The table gives common examples which are well known to have caused signs and symptoms. Most of these have been well studied and documented. However there are other additives and preservatives which may cause similar problems. In all cases, check the label carefully — if in doubt make a note of what substance you are using or avoid it.

hyperactive children was studied under controlled conditions. The results of these observations showed that the K-P diet did not improve significantly the behaviour of these children as a group and thus cast doubts on the association between the ingestion of food additives and hyperactivity. Some individual children did improve. Clearly more research is needed to find out which group of children responds to the dietary measures and which children may derive benefits from other measures. The group of hyperactive children who are 'over-senstitive' to additives is small in number, hence it can be difficult to uncover when large groups of children are studied. It is my impression that pre-school children are more affected than older children.

Table 6.8   Foods avoided in the K-P diet.

Fruit
>   Almonds
>   Apples
>   Apricots
>   Blackberries and cherries
>   Currants, grapes and raisins
>   Nectarines, oranges
>   Peaches, plums and prunes
>   Raspberries and strawberries

Vegetables and Vegetable Products
>   Margarine
>   Ice cream
>   Cereals and bread
>   Sweets and jellies, lozenges
>   Gum
>   Frankfurters
>   Jams
>   Tea
>   All soft drinks

Other
>   Oil of wintergreen
>   Toothpaste and mouth washes
>   Mint flavours
>   Perfumes
>   Medicines containing aspirin

If you contemplate using the K-P diet, or any other restriction diet, seek a referral to an expert because:

a. your child will require regular supervision from a trained dietitian.

b. the child will need regular medical supervision in order to determine whether the behaviour is improving or not and for how long should the diet be continued. It is my practice to offer the help of a local support group or the opportunity of discussing the problem with other parents.

OTHER TREATMENTS FOR THE HYPERACTIVE CHILD

Hyposensitization with food extracts

A number of workers have reported individual successful treatments with the administration of small amounts of food extracts which were placed under the tongue or injected under the skin. I have seen the methods in use while visiting the USA but have not been convinced of their efficacy and long-lasting benefits. The methods are not sound scientifically and would require vigorous assessments before they can be recommended. It should be remembered also that these procedures can be dangerous because they can cause severe, unforeseen, life threatening reactions.

The use of coffee

Some researchers have shown that caffeine, the stimulant present in coffee, altered beneficially the behaviour pattern of some hyperactive children. The way caffeine produces its effects is not known. There are various other stimulant drugs which found a place in the management of the hyperactive child who did not improve with other measures. Interestingly, when these drugs are used, the child's handwriting is usually first observed to improve considerably, and when the child is taken off the treatment, handwriting visibly deteriorates. This simple observation is sometimes used to judge the response to a particular drug.

Megavitamins

Occasionally a hyperactive child was noticed to improve when given large doses of vitamins. In view of the fact that some vitamins can cause serious and lasting harm to the child, any parents interested in this form of treatment are strongly advised to consult a qualified practitioner. I have no experience of this particular approach to management. A recent report from the USA (1984) did not find megavitamins of value in a group of hyperactive children, but others have found the treatment useful in a group of autistic children (vitamin B_6 — pyridoxine — was given). This is of great interest as the cause of autism remains unknown as well.

Behaviour therapy

The hyperactive child who does not have food allergy or an intolerance problem can benefit from the use of skilled techniques in behaviour modification, in basic teaching skills and in the alteration of his immediate environment which becomes suited to his particular style of learning. Facilities for such treatment methods are not widely available but are obtainable in some areas in the UK.

FOOD ALLERGY AND MIGRAINE
(from Greek, pain on one side of the head)

A number of children develop recurrent and severe bouts of headache for a variety of reasons. Some become allergic to foods such as cow's milk, cheeses, wheat, eggs, etc., some become intolerant to some foods, e.g. citrus fruit, or to food additives and preservatives, e.g. tartrazine. A few children develop symptoms because the foods they eat contain large amounts of naturally occurring pharmacological substances such as histamine or tyramine. Tyramine is a substance which is present normally in the human brain and it helps to release a hormone called nor-adrenaline. The function of nor-adrenaline is to increase the heartbeat and blood pressure and to act as a transmitter of impulses at nerve endings. It can be seen, therefore, how excessive amounts of foods containing tyramine can cause symptoms. The common foods which contain tyramine are some cheeses, tinned fish, broad beans, yeast extracts, chocolates, etc. Similar pharmacological substances (methylxantines) are present in various beverages such as tea, coffee and cola-drinks. Occasionally migraine attacks can be precipitated by inhaling some agents rather than by eating them, e.g. the odour of perfumes. Whatever the nature of the adverse reactions, symptoms occur between one and two hours or more after exposure, i.e. the reactions are delayed.

Tracy started to have recurrent headaches during the Christmas holidays when she was just over 9 years of age. The parents described the initial episodes quite vividly — Tracy started to complain of 'banging' pains in her head, mostly confined to the forehead and associated with seeing 'fuzzy' spots in front of her eyes and soon after feeling sick and vomiting. She felt rotten afterwards and preferred to lie down in her room with the curtains drawn. She had had few illnesses in the past apart from some eczema on her face and legs. The parents attributed Tracy's headaches to the excitement of Christmas and indeed she did appear to get better when the festivities were over — but not for long. A few weeks later the symptoms returned and became more frequent especially in the early evenings. Some of Tracy's headaches improved with aspirins and other similar measures. Since she did not appear to be 'growing out of them' she was referred to a specialist who found that Tracy's symptoms were due to over-indulgence of chocolates which contained one of the pharmacological substances causing the problem. Indeed Tracy herself confided that she would eat 'some sweets' on the way home from school — hence the explanation for evening symptoms.

Tracy's problem was solved and nothing was heard of her until she came again at 17 years of age. She did not eat any chocolate and yet her migraine returned. 'It is as bad as it always was,' she said, 'and sometimes terrible when I go out to see Edward — he is my boy friend.'

A detailed history and allergy tests revealed that Tracy became sensitive to orris root which is a special plant, the ingredients of which are used in the manufacture of many cosmetics, perfumes, lipstick, shampoos, hair sprays, scented soaps, etc. — and even scented candles! The offending culprit was the hair spray, some of the other toiletry products did not contain orris root.

Comment: Tracy's history shows how her attacks of migraine were caused by a food and later on by an inhalation of a different allergic substance. It also teaches us that months or even years of misery can be prevented by simple avoidance measures and without any other recourse to complicated treatments.

FOOD ALLERGY AND ECZEMA

See Chapter 7.

FOOD ALLERGY AND ASTHMA

See Chapter 11.

FOOD ALLERGY AND BED-WETTING

Bed-wetting is a little more common in boys than girls, and at about 5 years of age, at least 15 per cent of children continue to do so. Because of the frequency and familial nature of bed-wetting, a number of researchers have suggested that food allergy may be implicated as a cause in some children. This observation arose when a young allergic child started to wet the bed, while drinking large amounts of cow's milk, having become dry completely by 3 years of age. Others have incriminated eggs, wheat, corn and some fruits as the most common precipitating foods. There are no conclusive studies demonstrating that food allergy is an important cause of bed-wetting and similarly no studies are available regarding the efficacy of avoidance measures or the trials of specific elimination diets.

Other reports have also suggested that allergy can be responsible for some form of kidney diseases in young children, e.g. the nephrotic syndrome. Again the reports, mostly sporadic case-reports, are too few to base any objective judgements of beneficial efficacy.

Chapter 7

Skin Allergies

Skin disorders of one form or another are very common in infants and children. They may represent a true or a primary skin condition or they may constitute a 'mirror' of some underlying medical problem elsewhere in the body. Hence the first pre-requisite to a successful management of a skin disorder is an accurate diagnosis. Attempts at cavalier and instant skin labels by well-meaning but untrained persons is bad practice as it often leads to wrong treatment and confuses everybody around so that the parents lose confidence in any subsequent advice — especially a medical one.

It is worth remembering that:
- because we can actually observe the skin, we can follow the ups and downs of any condition from day to day.
- allergic skin conditions are not infectious, so let the child play with his peers, and thus avoid emotional upheavals which may affect the skin problem.
- however unsightly the skin may be now, eventually it will heal completely and without scars.
- be patient and follow sound advice — the majority of skin allergies respond well to an appropriate treatment.

ATOPIC DERMATITIS
(Eczema — to boil over, to break out i.e. to form vesicle)

The word eczema is just a description of changes in the skin. It is not really a diagnosis because some other medical diseases present as an eczema rash. The word dermatitis means the inflammation of the skin which is only one feature of this disorder. Thus, atopic dermatitis is an itching inflammatory skin condition, often associated with respiratory allergies (asthma, rhinitis). A positive family history of various allergies is often present, so when in doubt make sure that the word eczema is synonymous with atopic dermatitis — otherwise unnecessary suffering may result.

The characteristic features of atopic dermatitis are:

- it affects between 1 and 5 per cent of all children.
- 50-80 per cent of children will also have, or will develop, asthma or nasal allergies.
- 60-75 per cent of children will have one or both parents who have, or may have had, a similar condition in the past.
- 60-80 per cent of children when tested with skin sensitivity tests and/or blood radioallergosorbent tests (RAST) will show positive responses to various foods and allergens.
- 75-85 per cent of children have elevated levels of IgE antibody in their blood on initial testing.

> One day in January, Philip, aged 6 years, just as he was walking to school developed an angry, red rash on his hands and later on his forearms. At first the rash contained a mass of tiny and solid looking pimples which itched intensely. Philip scratched his hands and arms unmercifully so that by the time he got home later in the day his arms were full of crocks and fissures. The parents were told he developed 'eczema' and he was prescribed an ointment. Two months later and after the various ointments and medications did not appear to be beneficial, Philip's skin condition was thoroughly assessed. It was striking that at no time did Philip's rash contain any tiny blisters. Hence it was deduced that his skin condition was not eczema but had resulted from a form of skin contact — traced to an unusual pair of gloves! Simple advice was curative.

Comment: An accurate history forms a very good basis for an appropriate treatment.

Common features of atopic dermatitis

The appearance of the rash varies depending on the stage of the condition and the degree of involvement but the one symptom that persists at all times is moderate or severe itching. This observation is of fundamental importance as it helps in the management. If one applies some form of irritating substance to the skin of a child who does not have atopic dermatitis, he will

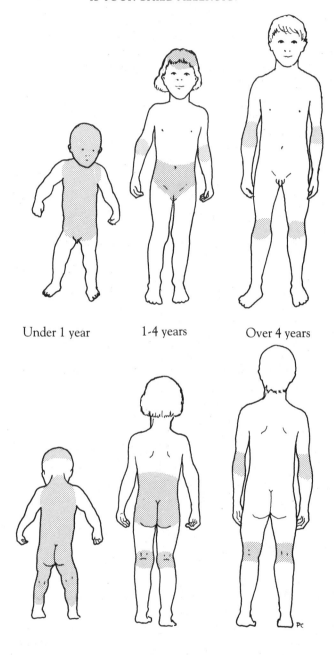

Under 1 year   1-4 years   Over 4 years

Figure 7.1   The sites of the body affected by atopic
dermatitis vary with age

demonstrate a very mild itching tendency only. The same substance applied to the skin of a child with atopic dermatitis will cause a very severe itching which will lead to rubbing and scratching of the skin and hence severe skin damage allowing skin bacteria to grow in the damaged areas. If any form of treatment interrupts the itch–scratch cycles, the condition will cause few problems for the child and his parents!

The infant

The condition appears at about 3-4 months of age, and involves often the scalp, face and other parts of the body. The rash looks red and angry and is full of tiny vesicles (blisters). In the majority of infants the rash will clear up completely by 3-5 years of age. Confusion can arise with:

- nappy rashes — these are due to the irritation of the skin by the ammonia released from the baby's urine on contact with the stools.
- seborrheic rash — these are the oily secretions made in the sebaceous glands of the skin and which act as a lubricant for hair and provide some protection against common skin bacteria. The sebaceous glands are found all over the body except on the palms of the hands and the soles of the feet.
- cradle cap — this is a seborrheic dermatitis of the scalp. There is hardly any itching and the condition clears up within the first two or three months of life.
- thrush skin infection — this is caused by a fungus called candida albicans. It is often first seen in the baby's mouth as tiny white spots on the tongue and inside the cheeks.

The child

The rash may appear for the first time or continue from infancy. It involves the flexural areas of the arms and legs, hands and feet. It often settles into a chronic and persistent form. When looked at carefully patches of crusty and flayed areas of skin can be seen in profusion. At times and for various reasons, acute exacerbations of the condition occur.
Confusion can arise with:

- contact dermatitis — from irritation or contact allergy
- scabies

What is the cause of atopic dermatitis?

The exact explanation remains to be found. Allergic and non-allergic causes can be of importance.

A high proportion of children have elevated IgE antibody levels which can rise and fall depending on the severity of the particular skin problem.

What makes the condition worse?

Anything that irritates the skin:
- wool
- nylon
- some soaps and bubble bath liquids
- detergents
- cosmetics
- perfumes
- animal hair and feathers
- house dust mites.

Anything that either causes excessive sweating or excessive dryness of the skin:
- hot, humid weather
- food allergy (milk, eggs, wheat, peanuts, chocolate)
- skin infections — by bacteria
- emotional stress — possibly because it stimulates the sweating-itching-scratching cycles.

Absolutely contra-indicated

Anti-smallpox vaccination of the child or any other member of the family where another child has atopic dermatitis. This is because s/he is liable to develop a most severe and often deadly virus skin infection. The 'cold sore' virus (recurs often on the lip) can also cause serious infection of other organs of the body when absorbed through the abraded skin — but treatment is now available. (Acyclovir — made by Wellcome Foundation).

How to manage atopic dermatitis

The following remarks are offered as a general guidance and apply to the majority of children.

• Hygiene
— Drying soaps should be avoided.
— Fatted soaps and shampoos are best, e.g. baby soap.
— Keep nails short to reduce the damage from scratching.

• Hot and cold weather
— Avoid over-dressing because it may cause excessive perspiration.
— Keep home temperatures at around 18°-20°C.
— In the bedroom use cotton sheets, light synthetic blankets or duvets.

• Clothing
— Cotton and soft synthetic materials are well tolerated by children.
— Other materials may irritate the skin.

• Bathing
Controversy exists regarding the benefits of frequent bathing. Frequent bathing can cause dryness of the skin, so in order to avoid this use emollient baths oils, i.e. agents that hydrate the skin surface and prevent evaporation of water through the skin. Useful ones are: Alpha keri bath oil (liquid paraffin 92%); Aveeno oilated (liquid paraffin 35%, oat protein 41%); Balneum (soya oil 85%); Oilatum emollient emulsion (liquid paraffin 64%, acetylated wool calcoliols 5%). Follow instructions carefully.

Emulsifying ointment baths are beneficial in children with severe and generalized skin conditions but are unnecessary when small areas of the skin are affected only.

Useful shampoos are: Those containing tar extracts, such as clinitar solution 2%; genisol liquid 2%; psoriderm (tar 2.5%, lecithin 0.3%), and T/GEL 2%. In some instances non-tar preparations may be more useful.

• School activities and play
Encourage the child to lead a normal life and to take part in sports and games. If the child is keen on swimming, explain that the chlorine in the water can cause skin irritation but that it can be prevented by the use of barrier creams. It is also of benefit to the child to take a bath containing one of the emolient bath oils afterwards.

Swimming in the sea does not present problems for the child

because the salty water can be helpful. Indeed the sea air is beneficial all round—high intensity ultraviolet light, cool, low humidity and dust free atmosphere. It is of practical interest that the Dead Sea water, which contains extremely high concentrations of mineral salts, has been found to be of benefit to some children with generalized atopic dermatitis. The claims that the water may contain 'curative' properties have not be scientifically substantiated.

- ## Hyposensitization (allergen injection treatment)
  In general, there is no sound evidence that this form of treatment is helpful. The treatment can be dangerous as the skin condition can deteriorate acutely immediately after an injection. Occasionally it may benefit a child who also has asthma due to respiratory allergies.

- ## Local skin applications
  Skin applications, whatever their nature and origin, do not influence the eventual outcome of atopic dermatitis. These treatments are of benefit for exacerbations but some may cause unpleasant side-effects. There are so many formulations that most parents (and doctors) get confused as to what preparations are best and when should they be applied. Should it be a lotion, a cream, an ointment, a paste, or even a gel?

Topical preparations (from Greek 'topos' — place)
Essentially the drug that is going to act on the skin has to be soluble in something which is free from contaminants and infective agents, and which should allow the acting drug to be released in adequate concentrations so as to obtain reasonable benefits over a period of time. Thus many substances contain some form of anti-bacterial agent and other ingredients that keep the formulation chemically bound together.

What to use and when?
The skin preparations are usually creams or ointments. A cream is an emulsion of oils in water. An ointment is a fairly thick, often greasy, formulation containing paraffin, lanolin, waxes, etc. At times it can be difficult to tell one from the other. Ointments, because of their nature, occlude the skin surface, allow good hydration of the skin surface, and good penetration of the active drug through the skin surface. They are useful if the skin is scaly, hard and dry. They can worsen an acute exacerbation, especially

when it is very weepy and ulcerated. In these instances a cream can be used or a wet dressing. If the child's face is affected, a cream should be used or a lotion, which is a watery preparation of the active agents, or even a gel—a watery formulation that disappears as it is rubbed into the skin. Greasy preparations should not be applied to the face, groins and arm pits.

When in doubt, check the contents of the preparation carefully and discuss further with your doctor.

Steroid skin preparations

These are incorporated into creams or ointments. The beneficial effects in atopic dermatitis are obtained by virtue of their anti-inflammatory activities. There are other effects as well.

The formulations are of different strengths and some should not be used in children. If given frequently and in excess for a long time, enough of the steroid can be absorbed through the skin to cause serious side effects such as:

- thinning of the skin
- striae of the skin
- excessive and characteristic weight gain (the child's appearance is like 'a lemon on a toothpick')
- stunting of growth
- mood changes
- poor response to stress, e.g. acute infection
- thinning of bones
- cataracts

A few examples of topical steroids and their relative strengths (or potencies) are given below. Before you use any preparation, always check its contents, especially as now many preparations can be bought at a chemist without a prescription, and discuss the matter with your doctor if in doubt.

Very potent or strong preparations (not advisable in children)
Beclomethasone diproprionate (Propaderm forte), 0.5 per cent; Clobetusol proprionate (Dermovate), 0.05 per cent; Flucinolone acetonide (Synalar forte), 0.2 per cent.

Moderately potent preparations
Beclomethasone diproprionate (Propaderm), concentration of 0.025 per cent; Bethamethasone valerate (Betnovate), concentration of 0.1 per cent; Clobetasone butyrate (Enmorate), concentration of 0.05 per cent; Flucinolone acetonide (Synalar), concentration of 0.025 per cent; Triamcinolone acetide (Adcortyle, Ledercort), concentration of 0.1 per cent.

Mildly potent or weak preparations
Fluocinolone acetide (Synalar), concentration of 0.0025 per
cent; Hydrocortisone (Efcortelar, Hydrocortisylate), concentration of 0.1-2.5 per cent.

The availability of these large numbers of topical steroid preparations, with their differing dose dilutions and pack sizes, can be
a hindrance rather than a help in the management of atopic
dermatitis. Short-lived successes with the most potent and
recently introduced preparations are usually widely reported and
lead to confusion. In addition, since it can be extremely difficult
to measure the actual amounts of application used in any day or in
any week, we cannot be certain how effective these treatments
really are.

A treatment I use is outlined below, and is offered as a
guideline. If you intend to use some of the principles, do discuss
them first with the child's doctor to ensure you are doing the procedures correctly and make any necessary changes in management
as the time goes on.

1. When the condition is fairly generalized and/or associated with
asthma or nasal allergies, try an exclusion diet (see p. 76).

2. If the child has patchy areas of rash, Hydrocortisone
(0.5-1.0 per cent) is applied twice daily to areas affected for four
days or until such time as the skin heals. Any further applications
are given intermittently for three days at a time.

3. If there is bacterial skin infection an appropriate antibiotic
taken by mouth is given for ten days.

4. Bathing with added emollient bath oils or an emulsifying oil
(this should be diluted first in very hot water and then added to the
bath water) is employed daily until skin healing occurs and then
twice weekly or more often if the child is a keen swimmer.

5. If there is a poor response to Hydrocortisone, one of the moderately strong steroid preparations can be used but for one to three
days only.

6. In order to reduce the intense itching and scratching cycle, an
antihistamine agent can be given before bedtime for five to
seven doses.

7. A number of older children may not respond to these measures, especially when they have a peculiar form of dermatitis
called nummular eczema (from the Latin 'nummus' — coin,
because the patch is round in appearance). A coal tar preparation
can be used beneficially. These preparations are best applied
during the autumn and winter months because the tar itself

may sensitize the child's skin to strong sunlight and cause undesirable reactions.

> *Susan was the second baby of parents who were perfectly well, although the mother used to have eczema as a child, and brother Tom, then aged 4 years, had had attacks of wheezy bronchitis. The mother was told that Tom was prone to bronchitis because he used to be bottle fed. Hence she was determined to breast feed Susan to avoid similar problems with her. She did so for a full five months, during which time Susan grew well. She was introduced to weaning foods and the other normal infant foods. Her progress was uneventful until about 7 months of age when she developed extensive and fairly severe atopic dermatitis — of face, trunk and chest and legs. She became miserable, difficult to settle and cried a great deal. Treatment with various topical agents was, on the whole, partially beneficial. At about 9 months of age she developed a recurrent cough and wheeze which responded poorly to various syrups used in the treatment of asthma. Both her asthma and her dermatitis cleared up following the introduction of a restriction diet. She remained on the diet until 18 months of age when various foods started to be introduced into her diet. She had a relapse when almost on a normal diet. It was impossible to find out to which foods or additives she might be intolerant. Nonetheless when Susan was re-commenced on her original restricted diet, her symptoms cleared up again. At the age of 2 years 6 months further attempts were made to liberalize her diet. Again the successes were short-lived. Finally, at the age of 4 years, Susan was able to tolerate most foods, but atopic dermatitis remained in the flexures of her elbows and knees. These patches responded to topical agents but flared from time to time. Her episodic asthma could be well controlled with bronchodilator agents. By the time she reached 10 years of age her asthma caused her few problems but the patches of atopic dermatitis persisted, although in a quiescent form requiring occasional topical treatments only.*

Comment: Susan's story demonstrates that breast feeding is beneficial in an allergic family. Perhaps a longer duration of breast feeding would have been better. The history shows also that various treatments may be required in the management of atopic dermatitis and how difficult it can be to pin-point the offending foods and when to relax the dietary measures.

• Allergy diets

Well over forty years ago an American doctor demonstrated that eating wheat flour caused severe atopic dermatitis in a child. Since that time many reports have appeared in the literature about the use of allergy diets, not only in atopic dermatitis, but also in various other disorders of infants and children.

The most common foods causing problems in about 90 per cent of allergic children are: eggs, milk, peanuts, wheat, soya flour, fish, chicken, pork.

About 30-40 per cent of children may have problems with two or more food ingredients — it is rare to find a child sensitive to four or more foods when challenged by mouth. In general, any child between 5 and 8 years of age, who responds poorly to skin treatments with the various preparations as outlined above, is very likely to be sensitive to some foods.

Depending on the age of the child and the foods involved, a restriction diet should be used for eight weeks, and it should be supervised by a trained children's dietitian. It is entirely wrong to commence any child on an elimination diet without having first assessed him very carefully. I have seen children with food hypersensitivity and atopic dermatitis who were referred to me because 'diets have failed'. In most instances, this was not the case. The elimination diets were often not carried out properly, the instructions which the parents were given were vague or non-existent, and the duration of dietary elimination very short, e.g. five days only.

Most diets for young infants are based on formula substitutes for cow's milk.

Table 7.1 Formula substitutes for cow's milk

Milk

Human	Best

Milk substitutes

Nutramigen	Hydrolysed protein of casein, sugar is sucrose
Pregestimil	Hydrolysed casein, contains glucose
Velatin	Soya protein, sugar is glucose
Sobee	Soya protein, sugar is sucrose

Other

Meat products, artificially manipulated mixtures.

CONTACT DERMATITIS

This is of two types:
- irritation of the skin by some substances such as detergents, solvents, alkali and acid solutions, etc.
- allergy when a reaction occurs between a chemical on the skin surface and the skin cells, so as to form an allergen which is then responsible for the reactions. The reactions are either acute (immediate) or they are delayed for hours or even days.

In both situations the affected patch of skin will look angry, red and weepy. There may be swelling of the skin and usually the lesion causes a certain degree of itching.

The parts of the body most commonly affected are hands, face, eyelids, neck, legs and thighs.

A guide illustrating the parts of the body affected and the possible agents responsible is shown in Table 7.2.

Table 7.2 Contact dermatitis – parts of the body affected and the possible agents responsible

Part of body	Possible Cause
Scalp	Shampoos, hair sprays
Eyelids	Cream, dyes
Face	Cosmetics
Ears	Metal frames, earrings
Nose	Paper tissues, nose drops
Lips	Lipstick
Neck	Cosmetics, dyes, metal
Armpits	Deodorants
Hands and arms	Gloves
Trunk	Undergarments, clothing
Thighs and legs	Clothing, stockings, socks
Feet	Shoes, dyes

The number of chemicals to which a child can be exposed in everyday life is limitless. For instance, a mother's perfume can contain between 500-1,000 substances, so it is hardly surprising that the infant can become sensitized to some of these, and other similar agents, during the first few years of life.

A carefully taken history and patch of skin testing will almost always identify the offending chemical or substance. The patch test consists of placing the suspected substance on an area of normal skin for 48-72 hours and holding it in place by an adhesive tape. The skin is then examined for redness, swelling and any vesicles or blisters. At times the child will remove the patch before 48 hours or so because of intense itching.

The treatment is fairly straightforward and consists of removing the responsible agents causing symptoms.

> *Tom was a fairly normal 14 year old boy who had two brothers who were also very well, and so were his parents. There was no history of any allergy in any members of the family. One day Tom's face was noticed to be intensely red, his eyelids became swollen and his face started to itch so that he started to scratch it all over. His mother wondered whether it could have been caused by the wind as Tom had walked home from school — about one kilometer away. Anyway, the rash cleared up within the next few hours and nothing new was observed until the following week. The rash appeared again when Tom arrived home from school — a week later to the day. Since the mother became concerned, Tom was seen by a specialist who found that once a week, on a Wednesday, Tom played football and then had a shower at school using a particular brand of soap, to which he had become allergic, but only on subsequent exposure of his skin to the sunlight. A patch test on his arm convinced Tom's doubting parents that he developed so-called photocontact dermatitis.*

Comment: Tom's problem was a little unusual and it required an accurate history which was supplied by him and his parents.

URTICARIA
(or Hives)

These are transient skin eruptions of wheals and round swellings associated with itching. They can last for a few minutes or for hours, but rarely over 48 hours. It is an extremely common condition in children (1-15 per cent) and occurs in two forms:

acute — occurs once or twice only, the episode lasts for a few hours and then clears up spontaneously.

chronic —recurrent episodes very few days or weeks. Some episodes may be associated with swelling of the tissues under the skin.

Some common causes of hives in children are:

- infections — bacteria
  - — viruses
  - — moulds
- parasites, e.g. threadworms
- foods, additives, preservatives
- drugs, e.g. antibiotics, aspirin
- insect bites, e.g. fleas
- contact substances, e.g. soap
- physical agents, e.g. extreme cold or heat, sunlight or after strenuous exercise
- emotions, e.g. excitement
- hereditary (rare) — because of the absence of a special enzyme, this condition can mimic urticaria and swelling of tissues. The diagnosis is easily established by performing a blood test, and specific treatment is available.

The cause of urticaria can be difficult to establish accurately. In some instances, the cause is self-evident and very little treatment is required. In other situations a full assessment is needed before the condition can be properly treated.

Jennifer was a 15 year old girl who had had asthma recurrently up to about 12 years of age. Most of her episodes were fairly well managed by her parents and at no time did she ever require an admission to hospital because of her asthma. Occasionally, she experienced breathlessness following jogging — a form of exercise on which she had become quite keen, especially as the activity allowed her to run through a beautiful park. She knew that if she took a bronchodilator before any of these prolonged jogging bouts she would not become compromised by cough and wheeze, and indeed she always ensured that a bronchodilator spray was at hand if required. One day, as soon as she started off, perhaps a minute or two had elapsed, Jennifer suddenly felt queer. A strange feeling of tiredness descended upon her, a red rash appeared on her face and then spread to her body, followed rapidly by an uncomfortable itch sensation. She began to panic as her head started to throb and her skin to perspire heavily. Soon her chest became tight and she started to gasp for breaths. In desperation she tried the spray but obtained little relief. She called for help from the nearest passer-by and was taken to the casualty department of the local hospital where she required urgent treatment for her shocked condition. She stopped jogging for a month but continued to play the occasional game of tennis. She felt well throughout and did not experience any cough or wheeze after any of these activities until one day when she started to play hockey. As during the first episode all the symptoms occurred suddenly, and again she required hospital treatment. Jennifer's investigations showed that she developed acute urticaria provoked by exercise in association with eating a meal containing sea foods. Measures were taken to prevent any more episodes and none occurred for the next four years.

Comment: Exercise itself can occasionally cause urticaria but most episodes appear to occur when a meal, usually of fish and seafoods, is eaten beforehand. The exact way these factors operate together is unknown. Prolonged exercise (of five to ten minutes duration) causes asthma after the exercise is completed, whereas in Jennifer's case the symptoms and signs of shock occurred almost immediately when the exercise was started. This is the pointer to the correct explanation of the problem. It is most important to recognize this phenomenon because it can be life-threatening.

Chapter 8

Allergies of the Nose

Our knowledge of all the functions of the nose remains fairly obscure. The sense of smell is one of its primitive functions, and other important ones relate to heat regulation, the humidification of air which is breathed in, and the protection the nose gives against various germs. But we do know very little about how the various drugs and sprays affect the physiology of the nose, especially its secretions and the function of the cilia (from Latin, meaning eyelashes, these are the fine thread-like projections from the surface of each cell which move in a rhythmical way in one direction only and thus propel any secretion or debris along and upwards). The sinuses (air cavities in the cranial bones) communicate with the nose, but their full function remains undetermined as well. Despite these gaps in our knowledge, some definitive advances in our understanding of the function of these structures have occurred during the last twenty years.

Allergic disorders of the nose in infants and children are often mis-diagnosed as 'colds', 'infections', or more liberally as 'catarrh'. Any inflammatory process involving the mucous membrane that lines the nose is termed rhinitis (from the Greek, 'rhis' — the nose). Rhinitis is either acute or exists in a chronic form. The causes of rhinitis are:

acute — due to infections such as viruses or bacteria
— due to allergy
chronic — due to allergy which can be seasonal, e.g. pollens, or non-seasonal (also called perennial), or infections.
— due to physical agents, e.g. sudden changes in the temperature or irritation from cigarette smoke, due to anxiety, or caused by overuse of sprays and nose drops.

HOW COMMON IS ALLERGIC RHINITIS IN CHILDREN?

About 10-15 per cent of children will develop seasonal or non-seasonal allergic rhinitis before reaching adolescence. Allergic rhinitis due to grass pollens (hay fever in the old terminology, or now termed pollenosis) is a little more common in boys than girls, often starts at about 4-6 years of age and may persist for one or two seasons, the average being about eight seasons, sometimes as long as twenty five years. Every fifth child with pollenosis will develop asthma before adolescence. A number of children sensitive to grass pollens develop both immediate and late allergic nasal reactions. During the immediate or acute reaction which lasts for about an hour, the child sneezes on and off and has a clear discharge from his nose. About four to six hours later, the nose becomes blocked by thick secretions and may cause breathing discomfort especially in the infant or the pre-school child. Also some children persist with nasal symptoms even though the grass pollen season has finished. This phenomenon is due to the reduction in the allergic threshold of the linings of the nose so that other allergens, which normally would not cause problems, become operative and thus lead to the persistence of 'hay fever' symptoms.

HOW TO SUSPECT ACUTE ALLERGY

The child will have most of the following symptoms:

Common symptoms
— Sudden bouts of sneezing and itching of the nose
— Watery discharge from the nose
— Nose partly or completely obstructed, i.e. the child is unable to breathe through the nose
— Watery and itchy eyes

Additional symptoms
— Repetitive cough especially at night (it is due to the irritation

of mucus in the throat)
— Mouth breathing (due to obstruction of the nose)
— Heachaches
— Pain in the face
— Bouts of vomiting (due to swallowing a large amount of mucus)

The child's face often gives a clue to allergy diagnosis.
Look for:
— Allergic shiners (dark circles under the eyes)
— Transverse crease across the bridge of the nose due to constant rubbing upwards of the itchy nose (some call it the 'allergic salute')
— Peculiar nose and mouth grimacing gestures to relieve the intense itching of the nose

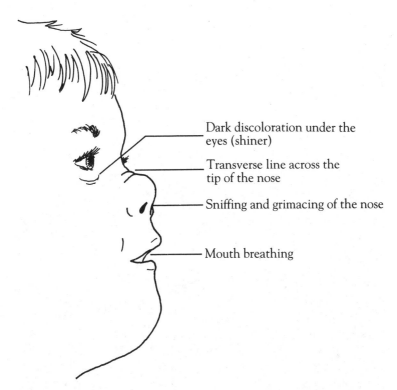

Dark discoloration under the eyes (shiner)

Transverse line across the tip of the nose

Sniffing and grimacing of the nose

Mouth breathing

(*Reproduced from Allergy in Children, J A Kuzemko, Pitman Medical, 1978*)

Figure 8.1   Some facial characteristics of allergy

ALLERGIC RHINITIS

The condition is caused by the reaction between IgE antibodies and the allergens on the surface of the mast cells (see Chapter 3) in the mucus membrane of the nose.

John Bostock (1773-1846), who himself suffered from nasal allergies, described the symptoms of seasonal allergic rhinitis as being due to 'the effluvium of the new hay' — i.e. hay fever. Some years later, Charles Blackley (1820-1900) established that the cause of 'hay fever' was not hay but was due to grass pollen allergy. Seasonal rhinitis has many causes — as a general rule, tree pollens are responsible for symptoms in the early spring, grass pollens in early and mid summer and weed pollens in late summer and early autumn. Some moulds can cause symptoms during the summer months as well.

Figure 8.2   What pollens look like

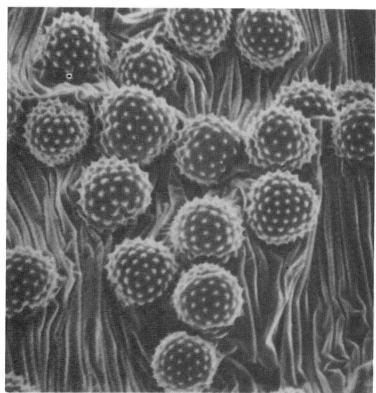

Perennial allergic rhinitis is caused most commonly by animal danders, house dust and the house dust mite, moulds and feathers.

HOW CAN I BE SURE IT IS ALLERGY?

A carefully taken history is often a pointer to an accurate diagnosis which can be confirmed as follows:

Skin tests with the specific allergens as suggested by the history. In this test a tiny drop of the allergen, diluted about a thousandfold, is placed on the skin, which is then scratched or punctured very gently with a small needle. The test is virtually painless and rarely upsets children. The skin test is positive when a wheal, accompanied by a surrounding flare, appears within ten to fifteen minutes and fades within the next hour or so. Occasionally the reaction may reappear four to six hours later.

Blood test — a small sample of the child's blood is taken and assayed for specific IgE antibodies. (The radioallergosorbent test or RAST.) The test is expensive but at times useful.

Other tests — there are other specialized tests which are used in research work and which have no place in every day practice, e.g. challenging the nose with allergens in order to produce symptoms.

ARE THERE ANY COMPLICATIONS OF ALLERGIC RHINITIS?

Yes, if the symptoms and signs persist for a long time the child may develop polyps (named after sea polyps which they resemble). These are fluid swellings of the linings of the nasal cavity and they protrude inwards causing obstruction to breathing so that the child becomes a perpetual mouth breather and becomes prone to infections of the sinuses and nose. When tested, the sense of smell is shown to be affected as well. The polyps vary in number and size and they look like 'grapes' i.e. smooth, solid, glistening and

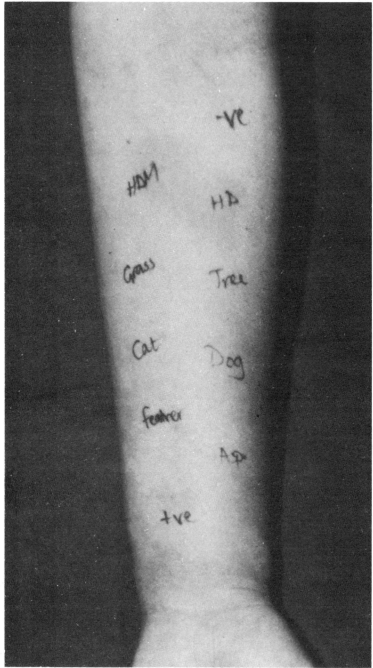

Figure 8.3   Testing for allergens

mobile. Nasal polyps are not peculiar to allergy and they can occur in association with other medical disorders. It is also worth remembering that children who develop nasal polyps may become sensitive to aspirin and aspirin-like products. These should be avoided, many are present in food additives. Check with your doctor.

MANAGEMENT OF NASAL ALLERGY

Avoidance measures

At times, and depending on the nature of the allergen, it may be difficult to avoid exposure. If the child suffers from grass pollen allergy, s/he should be advised to sleep with the bedroom windows closed during the pollen season, avoid playing in grass and s/he should stay indoors whenever the grass is being mown. If there is strong evidence of sensitivity to the house dust mite, you should try to take measures to reduce the population of the mite in the child's home, and especially in the bedroom. If you are going to employ avoidance measures, do the job properly. Half measures are useless. Your aim is to reduce the population of the house dust

Figure 8.4   Areas of the car that need to be cleaned

1 *Parcel shelf.* 2 *Lining.* 3 *Dashboard.* 4 *Carpet.* 5 *Mats.* 6 *Cushions.* 7 *Windows.* 8 *Area occupied by pets.*

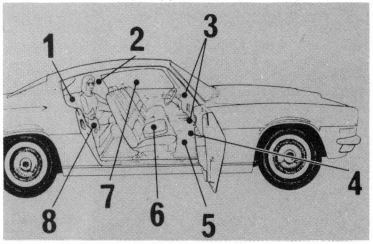

mite because to eradicate them completely is most probably impossible. So if you reduce the mite population you should reduce the signs and symptoms due to the allergy.

Here are some general guidelines:

Furniture — avoid stuffed or upholstered items. Best choose smooth wooden surfaces or plastic materials.

Materials — avoid woollen fabrics, heavy carpets, elaborate bed-spreads, mattresses and pillows made from animal hairs or containing feathers. Cotton and synthetic materials are best. Envelope the mattress in plastic and a dust proof cover containing a zip fastener. Air bedclothes outside in sunny weather.

Daily care — clean all surfaces in the bedroom with a slightly damp cloth. Vacuum the room and the house regularly, but when the child is at school or out at play, because such activity may spread dust particles about. Avoid collections of books and furry toys as they collect dust. Dust house plants daily. Keep the doors to the room closed. If you keep furry or feathered pets in the house take some positive action about what to do with them. Have a family conference. If in doubt seek advice. If the weather is warm, try to keep room humidity at about 50 per cent or less so as to reduce the chances of the mites multiplying. Ideally you should

Figure 8.5   Areas of a room that need cleaning
1 *Curtains.* 2 *Windows.* 3 *Cushions.* 4 *Air vents.* 5 *Bedding.* 6 *Bed.* 7 *Carpet.* 8 *Seating.* 9 *Doors.* 10 *Surfaces.* 11 *Soft toys.* 12 *Walls.* 13 *Blinds.*

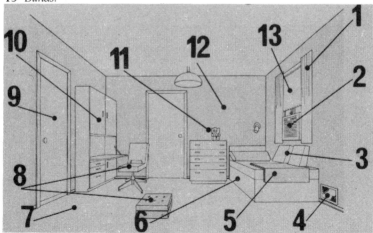

have air-conditioning; if not try a commercial air cleaner. Don't forget the car — keep the windows shut when driving — check the nature of the fabric of the seats.

Medical measures

The use of drugs given directly into the nose and acting on the fine blood vessels in the nose, making them less permeable to fluid (sympathomimetic agents)

The number of these agents is extensive. If used for prolonged length of time they may cause rebound phenomena, i.e. the vessels open up rather than become narrower so that the effects are the opposite to what was intended.

The use of antihistamine agents

Often useful if the symptoms are mild, and especially if there is a lot of itching. Unfortunately, many of these drugs can cause drowsiness and often dryness of the mouth, making the child excessively thirsty. Thus they are often best when given before bedtime. During the last few years, a new generation of antihistamines has been produced which has fewer side-effects. It is strongly advised that the antihistamine drugs should never be taken before any important tests or examinations. These agents produce beneficial effects within about 60 minutes and these effects last for up to three to six hours. With prolonged use the child may develop tolerance to the drug, i.e. it becomes ineffective.

The use of sodium cromoglycate

It is best when given before any exposure to the allergen. If given for grass pollen allergy, the drug should be started at least a week before the pollen season and continued for a week after the season is over. For other types of allergic rhinitis it should be given for about four to six weeks as beneficial effects may not be fully observed under two to three weeks of use. About 60 per cent of children with allergic rhinitis, of whatever cause, will derive worthwhile benefits. The drug is extremely safe and has practically no side-effects. It can be given as a spray, a powder or drops.

The use of steroids

The results of treatment are very similar to sodium cromoglycate, i.e. 60 per cent of children will derive useful benefits from repeated courses. It is given as a spray.

The use of immunotherapy (also called hyposensitization)

Leonard Noon, a physician, published a report in the medical journal *The Lancet* in 1911, demonstrating that injections of boiled timothy grass pollen extracts reduced the symptoms of 'hay fever' during the following season in a number of his patients. Despite vigorous research in this area, it is still not understood fully how this form of treatment really works but broad concepts are beginning to emerge.

During immunotherapy, i.e. injections of certain dilutions of allergen extracts over a period of time, the body develops a response to this stimulation by producing a specific type of antibody called a blocking antibody or IgG. These antibodies react with the allergens but they do not lead to the sensitization of the mast cells and the release of the various chemical mediators as happens when the specific IgE antibody is involved in the reactions. Undoubtedly other immunological changes occur and some of these are beginning to assume practical importance.

The composition and the dosages of the various allergen extracts have undergone changes during the last few years, mainly to ensure accuracy, potency, and purity, so as to allow better responses for treatments and the reduction of side-effects. Some of these side-effects can be quite serious and life-threatening. Thus the course of injections should be given only by a qualified doctor where facilities for emergency treatment for shock are available. The Committee on the Safety of Medicines reported in October 1986, that in the UK, since 1957, 26 individuals (adults and children) have died from the shock caused by these desensitizing vaccines. There were 11 deaths since 1980. They strongly advise that patients should be kept under medical observation for at least two hours after treatment and that there should be full facilities for 'cardio-respiratory resuscitation'.

Is immunotherapy worthwhile?

It depends for which particular condition it is used, (for asthma see p. 114).

It is most risky in any child under 6 years of age. If the child has proven grass pollen or house dust mite allergy, which has not improved significantly after a fair trial of the various measures outlined above, then this method of treatment should be considered. In general, about 60-75 per cent of children with seasonal allergic rhinitis will obtain worthwhile benefits during the subsequent one to three seasons, or even longer. One cannot predict which child will or will not improve. The results with non-seasonal allergic rhinitis are less impressive and often the courses of treatment have to be given for a long time.

> *Matthew had had asthma for many years. It was fairly well controlled on some preventive drugs and bronchodilators which he took by inhalation from time to time. When he reached the age of 8 years he developed grass pollen induced allergic rhinitis. Matthew's parents tried various remedies but with partial success only. The following pollen season which was very cold, rainy and windy, he suffered hardly at all. By the time he reached twelve years of age he could get by with the use of various nasal sprays and drops. At 15 years he had his worst time: by early June he developed a severe bout of asthma which brought him to hospital, and throughout this particular summer he had recurrent bouts of asthma and allergic rhinitis. Both the conditions subsided by early autumn. Since Matthew was due to take 'O' level examinations the following year he and his parents sought advice regarding the management of the next pollen season. Clearly, Matthew had not obtained any prolonged worthwhile benefits from allergen avoidance and the use of drugs. During the winter months a series of grass pollen injections was given, containing extracts of twelve varieties of British grasses, and from the beginning of May to make doubly sure, preventive drugs were given daily. Despite the high pollen counts in late June and early July of that year, and the anxiety associated with the examinations, Matthew did not develop any symptoms, although on one occasion he required extra doses of bronchodilators for his asthma. Similar worries occurred a year or so later when he was due to take his 'A' level examinations. From the winter of that year he was given booster doses of the grass pollen extracts. Again he had an uneventful grass pollen season. During his first summer at Agricultural College the symptoms of grass allergy returned, but abated again during the subsequent season.*

Comment: Every child's problem is different and is best considered on its merit. It is possible that Matthew could have done equally well with a course of oral steroids, or even an injection (or injections) of long-lasting steroids — just to cover him for the examinations. This was considered but it was decided to keep the form of treatment in abeyance should he fail to improve on the standard treatments. The case history demonstrates also how unpredictable the British pollen season can be!

When to consider the removal of tonsils and adenoids in the allergic child

The tonsils and adenoids contain important immunoglobulins which protect the child against bacterial infections. If these organs are removed, the release of these antibodies into the throat is very much reduced and may account for the recurrent throat infections which some children get following the operation. The long-term benefits of removing tonsils and adenoids remain a matter of considerable controversy.

Tonsils and adenoids often become enlarged in children with allergic rhinitis, but their size diminishes rapidly once the allergy is treated adequately. Little is gained from the removal of these organs in allergic children. However, if the child gets recurrent attacks of tonsillitis and ear infections, associated with a certain degree of deafness, or he develops a persistent glue ear (see p. 93) then the benefits of surgery are most welcome. In general, before surgery is considered it is worth thinking of allergy, because without doubt its management will be of greater and more lasting value than surgery.

Chapter 9

Allergies of the Ears

The ears may be affected by allergy in three ways.

1. The external ear can be involved in contact dermatitis (p. 77) In babies it is due usually to some soaps or a direct contact with animal pets. In the older child the allergy is caused by metal objects, such as earrings and spectacles, or cosmetics and hair sprays. Occasionally, the dermatitis can result from a prolonged use of ear drops — these are of little value in children and it is best not to use them.

2. The allergy can be a part of atopic dermatitis involving other parts of the body (p. 66).

3. The allergy can involve the middle ear. In the human, a tube (called the Eustachian tube after an Italian anatomist of the sixteenth century, Bartolomeo Eustachio) connects the middle ear with the throat and equalizes the pressures between the two sides of the eardrum.

In some children with nasal allergies a very thick fluid accumulates in the tube, causing obstruction and thus a degree of deafness.

Boys are twice as likely to be affected as girls, between 2-6 years of age. The condition is most common in the winter and spring months. In the majority of children there will be a history of other allergies.

The most common allergies are:
— *foods* such as eggs, chocolate, wheat and corn,
— *inhalants* such as house dust, the house dust mite and grass
  pollens.

> *Joyce, aged 8 years, had had asthma attacks from the age
> of 3. Her mother developed eczema when a baby and then
> had occasional attacks of asthma. Joyce's asthma
> considerably improved with various forms of treatment so*

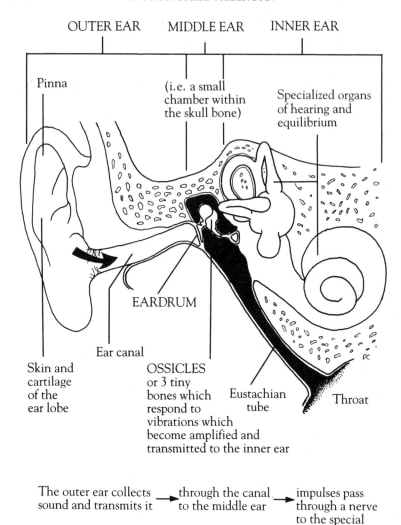

The outer ear collects sound and transmits it ⟶ through the canal to the middle ear ⟶ impulses pass through a nerve to the special centres in the brain

Figure 9.1   The structure of the ear

that she could play and enjoy herself, provided she took occasional doses of anti-asthmatic drugs. She had always been a happy and well-adjusted child, until early spring of the following year when her teachers commented that she had become 'moody, lacked concentration and appeared withdrawn'. She appeared jaded at home and would hardly ever watch her favourite programmes on the TV — she *preferred to be left alone. Joyce's parents tried all sorts of simple remedies but to no avail. A friend suggested dyslexia 'because of her lack of concentration and moodiness'. She was, therefore, taken to a psychologist who felt that she 'had a tendency to dyslexia' but was of normal intelligence. So remedial teaching was instituted. However, she did not improve as expected. A full assessment suggested that Joyce had developed 'glue ear' and hence conductive deafness, i.e. difficulties in hearing low-pitched sounds. The diagnosis was confirmed by an audiogram. The fluid aspirated from Joyce's ear had high IgE levels but the exact nature of the allergy remained a mystery. A simple surgical procedure allowed adequate drainage of her ears, and further anti-allergic measures prevented subsequent occurrences of tubes becoming blocked off with secretions. Within weeks Joyce became her happy self again. Her mother commented that the first thing Joyce said when she came home from hospital was, 'Why is the TV so loud?'*

Comment: Chronic ear problems are fairly common in allergic children with rhinitis or asthma. It is worth considering partial deafness when the child's school performance abruptly deteriorates. There may be other explanations for such a behaviour — hence referral to an experienced doctor should be made.

HOW CAN THIS CONDITION BE SUSPECTED?

The young child appears hard of hearing, having been previously quite well — s/he may start to play his music louder, or turn up the TV sound, or you appear constantly to be shouting at him/her! At times, the teacher or the neighbour may make comments that s/he 'appears not to notice' or 'lives in a world of his/her own' or 's/he does not concentrate'.

An older child may complain of buzzing in his/her ears, or that his/her voice is sounding like an echo, or that his/her ears seem to be constantly 'popping'.

WHAT SHOULD BE DONE?

If a degree of deafness is suspected you should see the child's doctor straight away. He may reassure you as to the likely cause, or ask for a special hearing test. The various allergy tests can be performed if clinically indicated. Treatment depends on the findings at the actual time of the examination.

INNER EAR SYMPTOMS

Vertigo (a sensation of abnormal motion often described as dizziness by children), tinnitus (hissing in the ears), and some impaired hearing are part of the so-called Menière's disease of adults (after Prosper Menière, a French physician who described the condition originally). However, allergy especially to foods can occasionally cause similar symptoms in older children. The condition improves rapidly following efficient treatment of the underlying allergy. It is important to bear such a possibility in mind in any child who develops vertigo and/or tinnitus.

Chapter 10

Allergies of the Eyes

The eye may be involved in allergic reactions in a variety of ways:
- as a part of the food allergy syndrome (p. 64)
- the eyelid can be affected by:
  — contact dermatitis (p. 77) e.g. from cosmetics (Table 10.1)
  — hives (p. 78)
- the conjunctiva can be affected by:
  — allergic rhinitis (p. 84)
  — hives

Table 10.1 Some common contact allergies of the eyelids

	Allergic substance
Perfumes	Almond oil
	Canada balsam
	Clove oil
	Jasmine oil
	Lemon oil
	Orris oil
Hair preparations	Dyes e.g. with lanolin, salicylic acid, etc.
Lipsticks	Eosin dyes, castor oil
Nail polish	Alkyd resins
Face creams	Borax
	Lanolin
	Salicylic acid
Face antiseptics	Phenol, benzoid and boric acids
Toothpaste	Dyes and preservatives

When the eyes are exposed to allergic reactions, they become rapidly swollen because the supporting tissues around the orbit of the eye are fairly loose and elastic so that any swelling is forced to push it forwards.

ALLERGY TO THE CONJUNCTIVA

Allergic reactions within the conjunctiva occur as a part of any form of allergic rhinitis — be it seasonal or non-seasonal. The first symptom is usually intense and intolerable itching of the eyes which the child tends to rub vigorously in order to relieve the discomfort. Such an action adds further injury to the already damaged membrane linings so that the swelling increases in size. When looked at, the eyes are intensely red, swollen and discharge a clear, water-like fluid. During springtime a specific type of conjunctivitis can occur. It is called vernal conjunctivitis (from the Latin 'vernalis' — spring). In this condition the conjunctiva is severely involved between May and June of each year. It occurs more often in boys than girls and especially in those children who suffer from other allergic disorders.

The exact causes of the condition remain to be determined. It is most important to recognize its existence because, untreated, some structures of the eye may become damaged permanently by, for example, ulcers of the cornea or scars in the conjunctiva. The most common causes in children are associated with grass pollens, house dust, various types of food allergens, and in adolescents it may be caused by wearing contact lenses. In this situation the itching of the eyes is often less severe than when the eyes are affected directly by some form of allergy.

Ben, aged 11 years, had had asthma and eczema for most of his life. He required regular treatments for both conditions, and on the whole managed to get by without having to be admitted to his local hospital with severe exacerbations of either condition. Certainly he noticed a definite improvement in his asthma by around 10 years of age so that the cold winter days which had prevented him from playing games at school were no longer a serious problem. Ben's father had had eczema most of his life and so did Ben's uncle. His sister remained healthy throughout her childhood.

Ben's twelfth birthday, which fell on the last day of May, was a particularly memorable affair — he felt in top form, many friends came to his party and it was a hot, almost summer-like day so that he and his friends could enjoy pursuits in the garden looking for 'the hidden treasure'.

A few days later, Ben woke up with painful eyes — he had been scratching the right eye through the night because 'it drove him mad'. The itching had become intense, his eyes congested and suffused, and there was a thick and discoloured discharge from his eyes. The examination of the eyes demonstrated the typical features of vernal conjunctivitis and a great deal of damage to Ben's eye linings because of the vigour with which he rubbed his itchy eyes to relieve the most severe discomfort. Applying ice cubes to Ben's eyes was soothing immediately, and further measures with steroids, sodium cromoglycate and antihistamine agents helped him to relieve the symptoms every year for the subsequent six seasons at which point the condition abated suddenly. There were no further recurrences during the next three years.

Comment: Vernal conjunctivitis is uncommon but when it does occur it is a most disabling condition which requires vigorous treatment and a great deal of support and understanding. It is more common in boys than girls, occurs in children who usually have other allergies, and tends to run a course of between five to ten years or so. What the exact nature of the allergy is remains undetermined — high levels of histamine are often present in tears obtained during an acute exacerbation.

If the condition is suspected (beware of intolerable itching of the eye!) a careful examination of the upper eyelid conjunctiva will confirm the diagnosis. Various remedies have been used in the management of this condition.

- steroid eye drops — make sure these are given correctly
- sodium cromoglycate drops
- cold compresses
- aspirin — given by mouth, and often. The beneficial effects are due to the effects on prostaglandins
- domicile in a cool climate — often helpful

There is a tendency, whatever treatments are used, for this condition to improve spontaneously after many years.

Chapter 11

Asthma

The word asthma is derived from Greek, and it means literally 'to breathe hard' or 'to pant'. Thus it is a descriptive word. Despite the fact that asthma has been afflicting mankind since time immemorial, the knowledge about its exact causes and the way these operate to produce symptoms and signs remains poorly understood.

Asthma is: a condition which causes recurrent narrowing of the breathing tubes which can improve completely with some form of treatment, or spontaneously, i.e. without any treatment.

Asthma runs in families. This means that it is inherited in some way, but the nature of such inheritance is still unknown. Whatever these inherited factors may be, it is the environment, i.e. the place where the child resides, that plays a most important role in provoking attacks of asthma. Some of these triggering factors are well understood but others remain to be worked out in detail.

Some common trigger factors of asthma are:
- cold air
- allergy, e.g. inhaled or eaten
- irritants, e.g. dust, fumes, tobacco smoke
- exercise
- virus infections of the upper respiratory tract ('colds')
- emotion, e.g. anger, laughter
- drugs, e.g. aspirin
- foods, e.g. some specific food may release potent pharmacological substances, e.g. red wine

MECHANISMS OF ASTHMA

There have been various scientific explanations how these

triggering factors actually cause the symptoms of asthma, but none has explained fully all the pathological features of asthma.

It is most likely that asthma is caused by a number of mechanisms, and possibly most of these are inter-related.

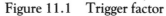

Figure 11.1   Trigger factor

Direct action
e.g. allergy

Indirect action
e.g. nervous
pathway

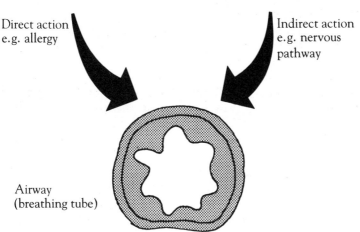

Airway
(breathing tube)

For instance, if a child is allergic to a specific allergen, the reactions will be produced by the effects of Type I hypersensitivity (see p. 24). On the other hand, an irritating substance will produce effects by a reflex action, i.e. the message from the airway is transmitted along a specialized nerve to the brain, in response to which another message is passed on to cause the airways to narrow, e.g. by constriction of the muscle and to release the airway's secretions within the tubes. No doubt there are other pathways which remain unknown.

In every human, the airways have the capacity to widen and constrict depending on the stimulus. In the child with asthma, this capacity for airway dilatation (widening) and constriction (narrowing) is considerably exaggerated. In other words, the same stimulus applied to a child without asthma may cause very slight response only, whereas in the asthmatic individual the response will be significantly magnified. This feature, which is called **the hyper-reactivity of the airways**, is a most characteristic finding in asthmatic children.

A large number of cells have been observed in the lungs of people dying from asthma. Hence many of these have been studied in detail in order to determine their particular role in the causation of asthma.

Some types of cells involved in asthma

- mast cells
- eosinophils
- neutrophils
- macrophages
- platelets
- epithelial cells

Damage to these cells, either because of allergy or some other stimulating factor, can be associated with release of potent

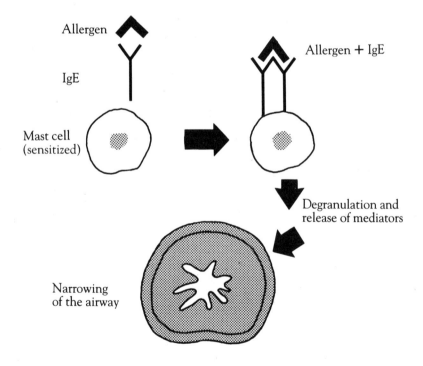

Figure 11.2   Type 1 hypersensitivity reaction within the airways

pharmacological substances, which in turn act on the airways, making them considerably narrow to the air-flow, i.e. the individual will experience breathing difficulties. This chain of events can best be illustrated by the damage to the *mast cells*. These specialized cells are abundant in the airways — and are present in all other organs except the brain. They contain histamine and other substances. A very high proportion of children with asthma (some estimate at least 90 per cent) are allergic to various substances so that they produce IgE antibodies (see p. 23) which bind specifically to the mast cells. If the child is repeatedly exposed to the same allergens, a cross-linking with the cell-bound IgE occurs and leads to the damage of the cell membrane and the release of a number of pharmacological mediators.

The way the various mechanisms operate is less clear, but there is little doubt that damage to these cells is directly involved both in causing asthma and also the state of hyper-reactivity. A great deal of research is currently taking place on how this excessive responsiveness of the airways could be reduced, and how one could prevent Type I hypersensitivity reactions from occurring. Some definite advances have been made and these will be discussed later.

WHAT HAPPENS DURING AN ATTACK OF ASTHMA?

Whatever the nature of the stimulus causing the narrowing of the breathing tubes, the child becomes acutely conscious of his/her breathing pattern, e.g. chest becomes tight. The narrowing of the airways causes an initial disturbance in the ventilation behaviour within the lungs so that less oxygen is transferred from the air to the tissues and the carbon dioxide content (the gas we exhale as part of the oxygen and carbon dioxide transport system) of the tissues becomes disturbed. The child then starts to breath quicker, possibly in response to the initial but slight disturbance in the carbon dioxide content, and also possibly because of anxiety or even infection. The result of breathing faster is that s/he gets rid of carbon dioxide very quickly but unfortunately cannot take more oxygen from the air (air contains about 21 per cent of oxygen). As the attack progresses the child takes less and less oxygen to the tissues, and eventually, once the tubes are almost obstructed by secretions, s/he starts to retain carbon dioxide as well. S/he is now pretty ill and requires urgent treatment with oxygen and other methods.

While all these events are occurring within the lungs, the child becomes progressively weaker. In order to maintain ventilation s/he has to work hard with the muscles of respiration, i.e. the diaphragm, the intercostal muscles, the abdominal muscles. These efforts require considerable energy, and since s/he is most unlikely to eat and drink adequately, s/he will utilize his/her body tissues, such as fat stores, for this purpose. An elevated temperature will add to the demands for extra fluids — but s/he may also start to vomit or even to have diarrhoea. This chain of events make the child dehydrated and acidotic. This clinical state has serious implications for the heart and circulation and other body tissues. Unless it is corrected quickly and efficiently, the child will enter a state of shock.

Table 11.3   The chain of events during the course of an acute attack of asthma

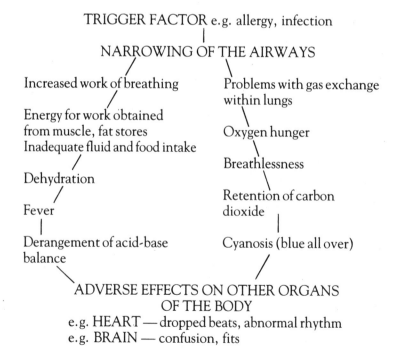

HOW COMMON IS CHILDHOOD ASTHMA?

In general, up to the age of 15 years:
- 2-3 per cent of boys have asthma
- 1-2 per cent of girls have asthma

In a study of school children, 5-15 years old, the distribution of allergic disorders was as in Figure 11.4.

Table 11.4   Allergic Disorders in Children (%)
(Peterborough, 1976)

	%
Asthma	4.9
Allergic and perennial rhinitis	8.2
Urticaria	5.7
Atopic dermatitis	1.2
Food allergy	1.6
Gastro-intestinal allergy	0.8
Others	0.6

At least 50 per cent of children who develop asthma, develop it by their fourth birthday and virtually all by their tenth.

At puberty, asthma in girls starts to predominate and by about 20 years of age twice as many women as men continue to have symptoms of asthma.

At puberty, 30-40 per cent of children become free of attacks of asthma, but some continue to have problems with exercise or after severe respiratory infections. By 30 years of age, only about 20-25 per cent of individuals remain symptom-free of asthma.

Many children who remain symptom-free for a long time, i.e. clinically perfectly well, can be shown on testing to retain the capacity of having hyper-reactive airways. Hence 'to outgrow' childhood asthma for good is uncommon.

About 35-45 children die every year from asthma in the UK.

WHEN TO SUSPECT ASTHMA

Any child who has
- a recurrent cough — often at night or after games

- recurrent wheezing — after 'colds', games, contact with animals. (Wheeze is a rasping or whistling sound especially prominent when the child breathes out)

should be considered to have developed asthma.

At other times there may be additional signs which your doctor will evaluate.

> *Martin, aged 6 years, had always been well until his parents moved to a new house — or so it appeared to them. The house was fairly old, a little damp, but Martin's parents were keen to modernize it as they went along. Martin was an only child; his father was a welder and mother a nursery teacher. None of them gave any history of asthma or other allergies, except that Martin's uncle who was in the Merchant Navy always developed a cough and wheeze when he returned home to North Wales. The first time the parents noticed that Martin was developing something was when they heard him coughing at night — with a rasping cough. At first they thought it was one of these 'colds' that everybody gets but since it carried on and on for days, and then weeks, they contacted a doctor who did not find anything abnormal. At this stage, a thorough assessment of Martin's condition was made. Tests revealed that he was allergic to a mould, usually found in bathrooms. Active measures were taken.*

Comment: Repetitive cough at night is a common sign of asthma. There are various causes which need thorough assessment.

Nigel's presentation of asthma was different to Martin's.

> *Nigel was a healthy well developed boy of 12 years of age who was a keen athlete and played every game that was available. He never had any problems whatsoever until one autumn day when during a cross country run he started to feel dizzy and weak and he found it difficult to breathe. He stopped for a while, got a little better and then continued again. But it was difficult. He completed the six mile course but felt pretty washed out. Lung tests showed that Nigel developed exercise induced asthma, but only after prolonged exercise; he coped very well with short games, and long distance swimming did not cause him breathing problems. He did not have any form of allergy.*

Comment: A long type of exercise is a common precipitating factor of asthma but it is the type of exercise which is of paramount importance. Free running is the worst. A very high proportion of children can be demonstrated to show this exercise effect which is due to inhalation of cold and unhumidified air. In virtually all children, exercise induced asthma can be prevented if the child takes a bronchodilator before any of the games s/he knows to cause breathing problems.

LUNG FUNCTION TESTS

There are various simple methods that the doctor can use to assess a child's respiratory function. Essentially most of these tests measure the amount of air a child can exhale out of his lungs with each breath. Thus, if s/he has asthma, i.e. the breathing tubes are a little or severely obstructed to the flow of air because of narrowing by muscle spasm and/or secretions, the test will show a reduction in the amount of air expelled with each forceful breath.

One such cheap but most useful instrument is the Peak Flow Meter and it is available in two ranges — one is suitable for children of 3 years and over, and the other can be used for older children and adolescents. The Peak Flow Meter can be used in many ways:

Figure 11.5   A Peak Flow Meter

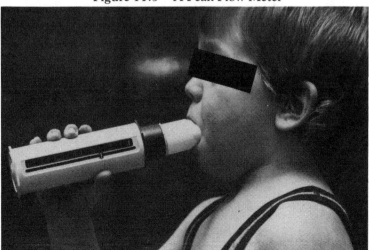

— to show any breathing problems after exercise
— to use at home (its best place) for demonstrating responses to any form of treatment or when to start to use treatments
— when new treatments are being tried
— to compare with a normal range of values in a child with similar height

Lisa, aged 9 years, had had many attacks of asthma since she started school. Every year she would be rushed to hospital on at least six or eight occasions because of the sudden deterioration of her asthma symptoms. The parents tried various forms of approach, but to no avail. Many investigations were performed by doctors which remained inconclusive. There was a general feeling that many of Lisa's attacks were produced by emotional factors, but the nature of these factors eluded doctors, psychiatrists and parents. Lisa was supplied with a Peak Flow Meter and recorded readings twice daily over a period of time. An analysis of the readings showed that she would be admitted to hospital when the readings were quite low but for two or three hours before there was a trend for the values to deteriorate. A practical treatment scheme was developed which offered maximum treatments at the first signs of

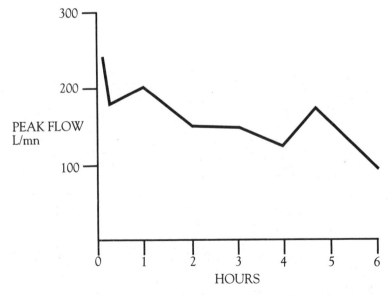

Figure 11.6   The practical use of peak flow meter

deterioration in Lisa's asthma. Her hospital admissions ceased and Lisa quickly taught herself when she required extra treatments.

Comment: It is often most useful to observe the child's progress over a period of time by using either a daily record card of symptoms or a simple instrument like the Peak Flow Meter. It is also worth exploring all possible precipitating factors of asthma.

There are many other specialized lung function tests which can be performed in hospitals or in research centres. Occasionally, such tests can be informative when used in association with the bronchial challenge tests, i.e. giving the child an allergen to inhale and then measuring the effects on the lung function changes over a specified period of time.

TO ESTABLISH A DIAGNOSIS OF ASTHMA

— needs a careful history of relevant symptoms.
— needs detailed family history, as in 75 per cent of cases there is a history of allergy.
— needs to thorough clinical examination of the child.
— may require additional tests:
   • daily record of symptoms for a period of time for accuracy and response to treatments
   • skin tests
   • blood tests for IgE (specific and total values)
   • lung function tests, e.g. Peak Flow Meter, either at home or in hospital, e.g. response to exercise, bronchial challenge tests.

WHAT AS A PARENT DO I NEED TO KNOW ABOUT ASTHMA?

Broadly speaking you need to know three things about asthma:
1. Basic understanding about asthma
2. How to recognise and treat an acute attack

3. The aims of long-term management.

Basic understanding about asthma

1. Try to learn the facts about asthma.
2. Consult your doctor and ask questions.
3. Write for further facts to:
   Asthma Society and Friends of the Asthma Research Council
   300 Upper Street
   London N1 2XX
   Telephone 01-226 2260

The Asthma Society is a national charitable organization which has about 141 branches all over the UK. The branches hold periodic meetings and lectures which are given by knowledgeable people about asthma and its management. It is worth enquiring whether a local branch exists where you live. Children are welcome to meetings and will benefit from sound advice. Through the Society's quarterly newsletter you will learn of advances in research and treatment.

There are a number of published short texts on asthma which you may find of interest. Contact your local library.

How to recognize and treat an acute attack

Once you have acquired basic knowledge about asthma, the recognition of an attack will not present a problem.

It is the duty of your medical practitioner to offer guidance and advice on emergency treatment. Remember that an acute attack of asthma is a medical emergency — so that you should have no reservations in contacting your doctor about your child. Minor attacks of asthma can be managed safely at home provided you know exactly what you are doing and are clear about the instructions given to you by your doctor. Severe attacks of asthma require admission to hospital because they are life-threatening.

Minor attacks of asthma at home can be treated with bronchodilators — given by mouth or a spray, syrup or tablet, injection, or through a nebulizer. In a very small child give the bronchodilator with the aid of a nebulizer solution.

The effect of the bronchodilator is to relax the muscle of the airways so that it 'opens up' or widens to allow easier breathing. There are many effective bronchodilators and there is little to choose among them. Some common bronchodilators are:

- Salbutamol (Ventolin) — most commonly used in the UK
- Terbutaline (Bricanyl)
- Fenoterol (Berotec)

Make sure how you should use these drugs when your child develops a new episode of asthma, i.e. when to start, how often to use and when to stop. It is best to write the instructions down.

A high proportion of children who develop attacks of asthma are treated with bronchodilators given through a nebulizer which is a very efficient method of administering the drug to the child's airways and enables a larger dose to be given to the airways.

A nebulizer is a chamber which converts the drug in the liquid form into an aerosol or cloud of particles. It depends on a physical principle allowing the creation of negative pressure in an area

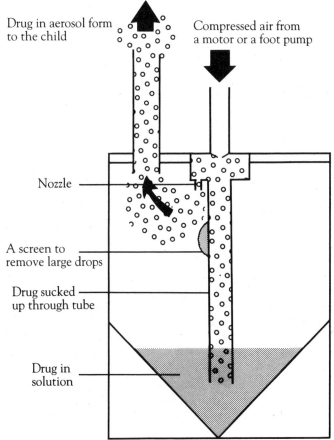

Figure 11.7   The principle of a nebulizer

when the air is pumped into it through a specialized nozzle. The solution, which is placed at the bottom of the nebulizer, is sucked up into this area and then released through an aperture in tiny droplets to the outlet and then by face mask or mouthpiece to the child. There are many nebulizers — some more efficient (and more expensive) than others. Seek your doctor's advice about the best buy, or consult the Asthma Society — they will offer helpful guidance — or you may obtain a nebulizer through the services of your local hospital. Remember that they need to be monitored and looked at from time to time to ensure that they are working satisfactorily. When you obtain a nebulizer ask about these facilities, because some pieces require replacement every few months, e.g. filters to avoid fungal contamination.

Some commonly used nebulizers are:

PORTANEB 50 (about £80, from Medic-aid Ltd, Hook Lane, Pagham, West Sussex, PO21 3PP).

INSPIRON (about £100, from Berol Ltd., Pennywell Industrial Estate, Sunderland, SR4 9EW).

MEDIX (about £70, from Medix Ltd., Medix House, Main Street, Catthorpe, Lutterworth, Leics., LE17 6DB). This firm makes an ultrasonic nebulizer also).

SINCLAIR ATMOLETTE (about £170, from Sinclair Medical Ltd., Burgh Road, Godalming, Surrey, GU7 2AB).

There are other efficient and durable nebulizers as well as foot pump compressors which can be useful when you are on holidays, e.g. camping abroad:

EASY-AIR (about £24, Cameron-Price Medical Division, 71 Melchett Road, Kings Norton, Birmingham, B30 3HL).

Apart from their use for the management of acute attacks of asthma, nebulizers can be used also to give other anti-asthma drugs for preventing attacks, e.g. sodium cromoglycate (Intal), and especially so in children under three years of age who experience difficulties in being able to take drugs by inhalation from other devices.

During the last few years, specialists treating children with asthma have become concerned about the unscrupulous use of nebulizers at home, the lack of their supervision and maintainance and the fear that over-zealous use may delay an urgent admission to hospital and thus lead to fatal consequences.

Thus you should be clear when and for how long you use the nebulizer during acute asthma. Some doctors, because of their fears, prefer your child to be brought to the Health Centre for the

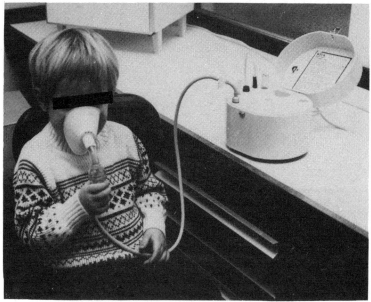

Figure 11.8   A child using a nebulizer

initial treatment and then will send your child home with the nebulizer to be continued for a short period of time.

At all times:

1. If the nebulizer treatment is not effective within 15 minutes, consult your doctor urgently on the telephone. If you cannot obtain immediate advice, take your child to the Accident and Emergency Department of your hospital and tell the duty doctor why you have done this.

2. Write down all instructions clearly, and the dose intervals.

3. Make sure your child's progress is reviewed within 24 hours.

4. Obtain your nebulizer through your doctor or your local hospital.

5. Make sure it is always in working order — clean daily with a solution of Milton — immerse for one hour, wash with water and then dry out.

6. Shake the nebulizer from time to time to make sure the mist is always coming through.

Severe attacks of asthma require hospital admission because:

— the child will need extra oxygen (even if s/he is given the same drug as you have given at home by a nebulizer).

— the child may require anti-asthma drugs and/or antibiotics (if infection is the trigger) being given through a vein.

— the child may require an intravenous drip to supply extra fluids to help with dehydration.

— s/he may require further tests e.g. X-ray of chest, blood tests.

Other drugs used in acute asthma are:

Iprapropium bromide (Atrovent) in a nebulizer

Aminophylline — given through a vein. It is often very effective.

THE USE OF STEROIDS IN ACUTE ASTHMA

These can be life-saving and often help to terminate an attack quickly, thus reducing the suffering from breathlessness to a minimum. These agents act by reducing the processes of inflammation from whatever cause within the lungs — thus they help the breathing tubes to become 'clean'. A short course of steroids given by mouth or injection does not cause any side-effects whatsoever. It is the long-term use of these drugs, often given indiscriminately, that is associated with adverse reactions. You should always question your doctor why they are being prescribed — there may be very good reasons to do so but you should be clear about them.

THE AIMS OF LONG TERM MANAGEMENT OF ASTHMA

The objectives are:

1. To plan how to treat exacerbations of asthma at home.

2. To decide what to do when asthma appears to be unresponsive to treatment.

3. To perform various tests which may help in planning treatment:

    — skin tests

    — blood tests

    — daily record card of symptoms

    — Peak Flow Meter measurements

4. To plan preventive measures:

    — avoidance of allergens or some food additives e.g. tartrazine, aspirin and similar products

    — diets (if food allergy is a factor)

— drug treatment
— psychotherapy or hypnotherapy
— breathing exercises may be helpful
— other approaches, if required, e.g. alternative medicine like acupuncture, homoeopathy, etc.
— immunotherapy (p. 90)

Some of these aspects of management have been discussed already, such as allergen avoidance (p. 87) and allergy diets (p. 74).

DRUGS USED IN THE PREVENTION OF ASTHMA

These are:
- sodium cromoglycate (Intal)
- steroid aerosols (Becotide, Bextasol, etc.)
- slow-release theophylline agents

It is best to give drugs for the treatment of asthma by inhalation because:

a. the dose given is very small
b. it reaches the site of action immediately
c. the side-effects are minimal

However, many children experience difficulties with the various canisters, i.e. their technique is poor so that virtually no drug reaches the lungs, it is merely swallowed. So at all times it is essential for parents to make absolutely sure that the child uses a correct technique.

The canisters can be:

Pressurized. The aerosol is ejected when compressed at an average speed of about 45-50 km per hour. If the technique is poor, the drug may get impacted in the back of the throat rather than being conducted to the airway.

Non-pressurized. Either a spinhaler — for the use of sodium cromoglycate. The child has to breathe in deeply so as to rotate the spinhaler's internal turbine rapidly in order to generate a cloud of fine particles. Or a rotahaler — for use with some bronchodilators and steroid drugs. The child has to breath in slowly to inhale the powder.

In view of the difficulties in taking anti-asthma drugs efficiently by inhalation, a number of modifications have been made to the

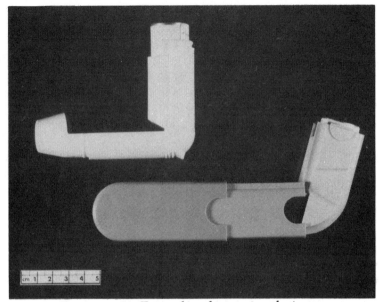

Figure 11.9   Examples of extension devices

Figure 11.10   A non-pressurized canister

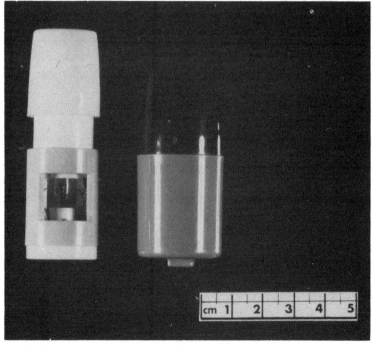

various canisters or large aerochambers so that the cloud of drug which is ejected from the aerosol can reduce its speed and thus allow better inhalation of the agent.

Some examples are:
— extension tubes and devices
— the nebuhaler
— the volumatic

It is absolutely essential that if your child is going to use any of the inhalation devices, that you and your child are given a demonstration of the correct technique to use. Not uncommonly the child and the parents give up using useful anti-asthma drugs because they do not know how to use these canisters properly.

Figure 11.11   A nebuhaler

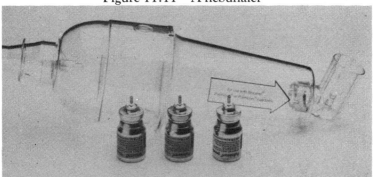

SODIUM CROMOGLYCATE

This agent has been used for treatment in the UK since 1968. It was obtained from a compound found in the seeds of a Middle Eastern plant, Ammi Visnaga, which has been used as a herbal remedy for many centuries. Its exact mode of action in asthma remains to be worked out fully. Between 60 and 70 per cent of children with asthma respond favourably to sodium cromoglycate. Its chief uses are:

• when asthma is poorly controlled with bronchodilators
• before prolonged exercise
• when a cough is the major symptom of asthma
• for some children who require frequent oral steroids

- as a long-term preventive agent so as to improve the child's airway hyper-reactivity. This effect is probably the most important

Sodium cromoglycate can be given as a powder, aerosol, and solution for use in a nebulizer. The use of nebulized sodium cromoglycate can be beneficial with infants who respond badly to other forms of treatment.

As with all the other drugs which are given by inhalation for asthma, either as an aerosol or in a powder form, about 10 per cent of the drug reaches the child's lungs — the rest is swallowed and excreted, unabsorbed, in the child's faeces (almost 90 per cent). Thus the technique of using inhalers for asthma is of fundamental importance. Follow the instructions very carefully. A practical demonstration of the method by a doctor or a nurse will be of great assistance.

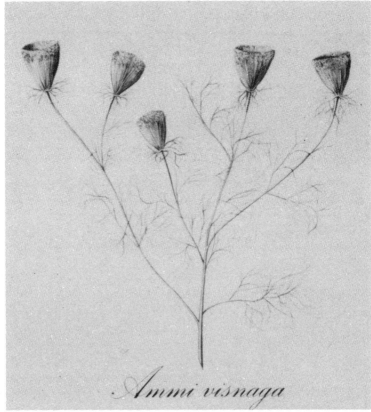

Figure 11.12 *Ammi visnaga,* **the plant from which sodium cromoglycate was discovered**

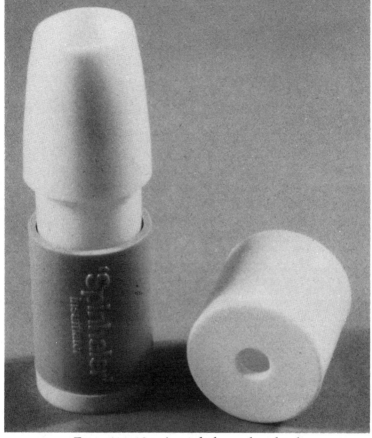

Figure 11.13   A spinhaler and a whistle

STEROID AEROSOLS

These agents were introduced for the treatment of asthma by inhalation during the early 1970s. Steroids were first used in medicine in the early 1950s especially in the treatment of rheumatoid arthritis and other conditions. Since then they have been studied in great depth so that, with careful use, side-

Aerosol deposition

Mouth (90-100%)

Stomach
(90%)

Lungs
(10% or less)

effects are now most uncommon. They act by damping down the inflammatory processes which are a part and parcel of persistent asthma. As with sodium cromoglycate and aerosol bronchodilators, about 10 per cent reaches the lungs from an aerosol so that a correct technique of inhalation is imperative.

Essentially there are four steps in the efficient use of pressurized aerosol inhalers:

1. Remove the cover from the mouthpiece and shake the inhaler.
2. Breathe out gently.
3. Place the mouthpiece in your mouth with your lips close around it, start to breathe in deeply but slowly pressing the metal canister downwards to release the powder and continue breathing in.
4. Remove the inhaler and hold your breath for as long as comfortable, i.e. about ten seconds.

Repeat the whole procedure if required.

Keep the mouthpiece and the body of the spinhaler clean by washing them with warm water twice weekly.

Your doctor will instruct you which steroid aerosol to use, how often and for how long you should take it.

Examples: Beclomethasone diproprionate (Becotide)
Betamethasone valerate (Bextasol)

THEOPHYLLINE PREPARATIONS

These agents have been used in the treatment of asthma since 1936. Caffeine, which is present in tea leaves and coffee seeds, and theophylline, which is also present in tea leaves and other 'soft drinks', are related compounds. Man has made beverages from the extracts of tea and coffee plants because of their stimulant actions on the central nervous system. The legend credits the discovery of coffee to a prior in the Middle East who noticed that goats which had eaten the berries of the coffee plant frisked and frolicked throughout the night instead of resting peacefully. Since the prior had to spend many a night praying (and usually falling asleep from time to time!) he picked the berries and made a beverage from them. The success of this experiment has been felt throughout the world ever since.

Despite its antiquity, the exact way the theophylline acts in asthma is not fully known — it is a bronchodilator, has some positive action on the diaphragm and other respiratory muscles and on the respiratory centre in the brain. However, the agents may act on other organs causing undesirable side-effects, e.g. on the heart causing palpitatións, on the stomach causing nausea or vomiting, on the central nervous system causing headaches and sleeplessness. Various factors affect their metabolism so that the doses require adjustments.

Figure 11.15   Factors affecting metabolism of theophylline

Lower dose needed
- infant under 1 year of age
- virus infection
- fever
- influenza immunization
- other drugs
  — Erythromycin

Higher dose needed
- child 1-7 years of age
- high protein foods
- other drugs
  — phenytoin
  (used for epilepsy)

Effective slow-release formulations of theophylline are available, which are slowly absorbed from the gastrointestinal tract so as to provide relatively steady concentrations throughout a 24-hour period.

Some common examples are:
- Neulin
- Phyllocontin
- Slo-phyllin
- Theo-dur
- Theograd
- Uniphyllin

(Check with your doctor for recent additions to the list).

There is little to choose between the various preparations. Most doctors check the adequacy of the theophylline dosage by estimating blood theophylline levels. This is a sure way of knowing the right dosage and it avoids undesirable side-effects. Most hospitals in the UK provide easily accessible facilities for the blood measurements.

BREATHING EXERCISES

The value of breathing exercises during an acute attack remains unresolved. If the child is able to relax with them and feels they are helpful, s/he should be encouraged to continue the exercises throughout the attack.

Many children derive subjective benefit from these exercises between attacks of asthma. The breathing exercises do help to teach the child how to use the muscles of breathing to the best advantage and thus also improve the child's physical fitness.

Thus breathing exercises:
- improve chest expansion
- tend to improve ventilation
- correct chest deformities, e.g. round shoulders

The principle of the breathing methods is to increase the child's intra-abdominal pressure so as to help to move the diaphragm high up in the chest — thus aiding breathing out.

There are some children with chronic asthma who dislike breathing exercises because they make them more breathless. Hence one should not impose them without a careful appraisal and discussion with the child.

PHYSICAL FITNESS EXERCISES

A planned physical education programme based on types of exercise is very beneficial for the asthmatic child. For instance, a three months course of intensive training, consisting of a one hour session two to four times a week, can improve the child's posture, increase fitness, reduce body fat and importantly, lead to a decrease in the symptoms of asthma and therefore a reduction in the use of medications.

A number of schemes have been evolved which consist essentially of graded physical activities of two to three months' duration so as to achieve a high level of fitness. These exercises do not change the underlying processes of asthma but they increase the efficiency of the muscles of the heart and circulation so that the child can perform well by utilizing less oxygen for these tasks. These exercises exert psychological benefits as well.

Prolonged and uninterrupted exercises of ten to fifteen minutes' duration or longer are tolerated badly by the asthmatic child. It is the inhalation of cold and unhumidified air that leads to the narrowing of the airways. In virtually all children, exercise induced asthma can be prevented by their making use of a bronchodilator beforehand.

ACUPUNCTURE

This is a traditional form of Chinese medicine which consists of puncturing the skin with a very fine needle at various specific points of the body. Acupuncture has been practised in China for at least 3,000 years and the practice was first brought to the attention of Europeans during the seventeenth century by a Dutchman called Willem Ten Rhyme (1683).

According to traditional Chinese medicine there are anatomical channels of the body — 12 main channels, each representing an organ. Energy passes through these channels and the points of acupuncture are situated on them so as to exert a maximum effect on the flow of the energy. A disease occurs when the balance between activity and passivity (called Yang and Yin) is seriously disturbed — thus by correcting the imbalance the patient can be restored to normal health.

The way acupuncture is helpful in some asthmatic children remains unresolved. The application of acupuncture needles to specific points in the child's back can be associated with widening or dilation of the airways — possibly through the effects on the autonomic nervous system. If practised by experienced medical practitioners, acupuncture is relatively free from any unwanted side-effects.

A list of qualified acupuncturists can be obtained from:
The British Acupuncture Association and Register
22 Hockley Road
Rayleigh
Essex SS6 8EB

HOMOEOPATHY

The essential principle of homoeopathic medicine is that 'like is treated by like' (the similia principle). That is, if a substance can cause disease it can also cure it or ameliorate it by the administration of the substance in various graded dosages. Homoeopathy has been practised since the days of Hippocrates (400 BC) but it was not until 1810 that the subject aroused considerable interest following the experiments of Samuel Hahnemann (1755-1843).

The benefits of the homoeopathic approach in childhood asthma remain to be medically proven. There are no published controlled studies to suggest that homoeopathy is superior to placebo. A recent study of homoeopathic potency in subjects with hay-fever suggested that there were benefits from that particular approach to the management. Also a trial of feverfew was beneficial in preventing attacks of migraine.

THE USE OF HERBAL MEDICINE IN ASTHMA AND OTHER ALLERGIES

The British Herbal Pharmacopoeia contains full descriptions of 240 herbs and their uses in treatment, but there are at least 1,500 herbal products which can be bought commercially. Many of these medicines are used for relatively minor and often self-limiting conditions, and little is known how efficacious and safe herbs really are because there are so few clinical trials. Some of the herbs, if improperly used, and for a long time, can cause serious side-effects. For instance, comfrey, which is used in the preparation of herbal teas, can lead to liver disorder, and chamomile, marigold and golden rod can cause severe anaphylactic reactions in children with allergies and asthma.

Thus, although herbal medicines are natural, they are not necessarily safe — the majority are harmless and some children may derive benefit from their careful use, but occasionally unexpected and serious toxicity can result. Also some herbal remedies may react together when the child is receiving drugs used on prescription — thus you should always ensure that it is safe to use them by consulting a qualified medical herbalist.

HYPNOTHERAPY

Hypnosis as a method of treatment of childhood asthma has been used for hundreds of years. Suggestion plays not an insignificant role in many medical treatments. In selected children with asthma the benefits of hypnotherapy are excellent. Similar beneficial results can be obtained also with family psychotherapy conducted by skilled practitioners.

Ruth was just over 10 years of age when first seen in the

special asthma clinic. The parents gave a detailed history of recurrent and severe attacks of asthma which commenced during the third year of life and which had continued ever since, every few weeks. Ruth required at least four or five hospital admissions every year because of the severity of attacks. She had been fully investigated by a number of experts, and various treatments and remedies were prescribed, which changed from time to time. There was no convincing family history of atopy or any other precipitating factors. Apart from asthma, Ruth was very fat because of the numerous courses of steroids which she required over the years and her school attendance record was abysmal so that she was well behind in her scholastic achievements. Since the conventional approach to the management of asthma failed, hypnotherapy sessions were commenced after a full discussion with parents and the child herself. The response after a number of sessions and a self-hypnosis scheme was remarkable. Ruth remained free from asthma attacks for nine months. Since then a number of repeated sessions were required and her drug management could be curtailed significantly. Within two years she shed her excess fat, made great strides in the classroom and was even selected for the school hockey team — a feat which would not have been contemplated even two years earlier. Her asthma improved further during puberty.

Comment: There is a definite place for hypnotherapy in selected children with asthma. The person treating the child with asthma should be the one employing hypnotherapy. One should be fully aware of its benefits and its limitations — it is a most useful adjunct to the management. At least four to six children are treated a year in a large specialized asthma clinic.

OTHER APPROACHES TO THE MANAGEMENT OF ASTHMA

The removal of the asthmatic child from the home and parents is considered by some to be a useful measure. The decision to admit a child to a special school for one or two years is an arbitrary one and depends on many factors — educational, residential, social, financial and emotional. Residential schooling for the child with asthma should be considered when there exist serious emotional problems in the family as a result of which the child's educational attainments become seriously impaired. It is essential to discuss all aspects with the parents, the child and the education authorities. In selected instances, residential schooling is of considerable benefit to the child and his asthma as well as the parents.

ASTHMA ASSOCIATED WITH HOBBIES

It has been known for many decades that inhalation of certain dusts, fumes and gases can cause asthma. With the advent of plastic materials during the last 40 years some children have been found to have developed asthma because of the inhalation of chemicals in the plastic materials, e.g. di-isocynates and acid anhydrides. Asthma as a result of recurrent exposure to various occupational agents is relatively common in adults but some children may develop similar problems if they handle various chemicals in the school laboratories, carpentry rooms, metal welding or photography.

Some common occupational agents which cause asthma.
- organic dyes
- dusts and grass extracts
- sterilizing agents
- metal fumes and salts
- organic chemicals — amines, acrylates, anhydrides, formaldehyde, isocyanates, etc.

The asthma symptoms result because of the Type I IgE mediated reactions in the majority of instances but in certain cases asthma occurs as a result of a non-specific irritant response. The best treatment is to remove the child from the environment associated with symptoms.

> Donald was perfectly well until he joined the senior school. His parents noticed that most Wednesday evenings he would start to cough, wheeze and 'splutter'. They ignored

the symptoms initially but when they persisted they sought a medical opinion. There was no family history of allergy, and indeed Donald's brother and sister were keen athletes and the father was a jogger. Tests showed that Donald had hyper-reactive airways but it was not clear what were the triggering factors. He was asked to keep a daily record card of symptoms and to use a Peak Flow Meter twice daily for 14 days. The readings confirmed the parents' story — Wednesday evening was the only time when Donald had asthma. Further inquiries revealed that Donald had started to help out in the photography department, and every Wednesday afternoon handled sheets of photographic paper. He developed asthma because the paper contained potassium chloroplatinate — a chemical which can be a cause of asthma.

Comment: Diligent search for the culprit is usually rewarding. Donald was advised regarding the handling of the photographic materials and every Wednesday took sodium cromoglycate which prevented further attacks.

Chapter 12

Anaphylaxis

The term anaphylaxis implies a severe and general allergic reaction, i.e. a reaction leading to a state of shock. The word was coined by two French doctors, P. Portier and C. Richet in 1902 — it literally means the opposite of 'protection'.

The sequence of events is as follows:

The child becomes exposed to the offending allergen to which s/he has been found to be sensitive previously. Within minutes, or occasionally an hour or so, the allergen reacts with the specific IgE antibodies which are bound to the mast cells. Thus a reaction occurs which stimulates the release from the cells of potent pharmacological substances acting on:

- the skin, i.e. a fulminating rash, tingling of skin, etc.
- the respiratory system, i.e. breathing problems, wheeze, etc.
- the gastrointestinal system, i.e. cramp in abdomen, diarrhoea, vomiting
- the heart and circulation, i.e. rapid pulse, acute fall in blood pressure, etc.

The severity of symptoms varies depending to what extent each of these organs is affected.

HOW COMMON IS ANAPHYLAXIS?

About two children out of ten million people get these reactions which are more common in children who have known allergies than in those without any allergic disorders.

The most common causes are:

- antibiotics — especially penicillin
- bee stings
- foods — fish, nuts, eggs

- extract of allergens used for immunotherapy
- horse serum
- reactions to radiographic contrast media

Some of these reactions are not due to allergy. They tend to occur more often in children with allergy and sensitive to iodine and shellfish.

There are some children who develop anaphylactoid reactions — and sometimes more than one or two — for reasons which remain obscure. Even the most careful investigations fail to find the exact cause. Fortunately the treatment is similar to that used for the anaphylaxis caused by known allergies and some children improve spontaneously with age.

There is also a group of children who develop anaphylaxis with exercise — usually following a seafood or fish meal.

> *Evelyn, a 14 year old girl with recurrent asthma, started to develop abdominal colic when she returned from school. Her mother did not become particularly concerned until Evelyn became violently sick, became feverish and started to complain bitterly that her abdominal pains had now shifted to the back. She was found to have an acute urinary tract infection which responded very well to an antibiotic. A few weeks later Evelyn experienced a similar episode. She was sent, therefore, to hospital for a special kidney X-ray requiring the injection of a dye through the vein in the arm. As soon as the injection was completed Evelyn started to feel flushed, hot, sweaty and felt her heart thumping away. She started to panic as she felt a dreadful sensation of being choked and having difficulties with breathing. The speed of the reactions was so quick that by the time a doctor arrived from the other side of the department, Evelyn was feeling dizzy and faint and became convinced she was dying. Emergency treatment was instituted and she recovered quickly and completely.*

Comment: Evelyn developed an anaphylactic reaction to the radiographic dye. These reactions are easily preventable if it is known by everyone that the child who requires some specialized tests is also an allergic individual. As a rule this information is requested before such procedures. Thus always volunteer to the doctor or nurse information about your child's present or past illnesses because it may be very relevant. A few years later Evelyn required a similar test again. A scheme of preventive treatment was instituted so that she did not develop adverse reactions to the dye — despite being terrified of the prospect!

WHAT CAN I DO?

Prevention is the best treatment.

The child should wear a bracelet (e.g. medic-alert) stating that s/he has developed an anaphylactic shock and to what agent — this is a useful precaution in case of an unexpected accident or other medical emergency.

It is useful to keep a syringe with adrenaline in your handbag and at home and school. (See p. 134)

The investigation and management of anaphylaxis requires supervision in an Allergy Clinic.

Chapter 13

Allergies to Bites and Stings

Fatal reactions to bee or wasp stings occur every year throughout the world. Egyptian hieroglyphics depict a lethal bee or wasp sting from which King Menes died in 2640 BC. Every summer in the UK five to seven deaths occur.

There are two ways in which the child develops an allergic reaction:

1. By the actual insect bite.
2. By inhaling the insect's emanations, i.e. what it produces.
   This happens in children who live near ponds, lakes or rivers. Most common culprits are aphids, moths or even allergy to cockroaches which can be caused by eating them as well!

BITING INSECTS

The most common are horse-flies, midges, bugs, mosquitoes, harvest mites and fleas. Some insects such as midges or mosquitoes, often cause multiple bites which are associated with severe itching of the area of skin affected.

The allergic reactions are usually urticarial rashes — with a raised central area. You can often see the opening of a bite if you use a magnifying glass. These rashes may persist for days or even weeks so that parents may not suspect that the rash was due to insect bites.

What to do

- Try to avoid them.
- Use calamine lotion, or occasionally, antihistamines.

STINGING INSECTS

There are a huge number of species of the order Hymenoptera but only four families are responsible for allergic reactions in humans. These are: honey-bees, hornets, wasps, and bumble-bees.

Other stinging insects which may cause allergic reactions are ants — especially the fire ant.

Table 13.1   Simple classification of common stinging insects

HYMENOPTERA

APIDAE		VESPIDAE	
HONEY-BEE (small, black and tan stripes, non-aggressive)	BUMBLE-BEE (noisy, yellow and black stripes, non-aggressive)	HORNET (yellow and white stripes) YELLOW JACKET (yellow and black stripes) – both very aggressive	WASP (thin-bodied, aggressive)

How do stings occur?

The egg-laying organ of the female bee, or wasp, etc., consists of two specialized appendages at the end of the abdomen. This organ is pointed sharply and contains the poison (or sting) which the insect can inject into its prey. Thus, only the females sting and most likely they sting in self-defence, although wasps can be aggressive! As a rule the female dies following the sting because during the process of stinging the appendage becomes dismembered completely.

The poison (or venom) of the Hymenoptera family contains various substances which are responsible for allergic reactions. Some of these identified fully are:
- histamine
- phospholipase
- hyaluronidase
- mellitin, etc.

The composition of the venom varies from one insect to another. For instance, the honey-bee venom contains noradrenaline, dopamine, apanin and mellitin, whereas hornet's venom contain a great amount of acetylcholine. The significance of the variations in composition of the venom is unknown.

About 50-100 micrograms of poison is injected each time a honey-bee stings. It has been estimated that 300-500 stings would be fatal to any adult person. However, I know of a bee-keeper who survived at least 1,000 stings! Hence there must be other and additional factors.

The allergic reactions responsible for symptoms are:

Local reaction at the site of the sting
Pain and swelling of the area within minutes of a sting. The area will remain tender and undurated for many days. An infection in the site can occur unless carefully managed.

General reaction, i.e. an anaphylaxis
It occurs in 0.2–1 per cent of stinging reactions. The reaction occurs within one hour of the sting and involves skin rash and respiratory difficulties, because of the rapid onset of swelling in the upper airway and spasm of the breathing tubes. A state of shock ensues very rapidly.

Atypical reaction
Hours or days after a sting, the child may develop a serum sickness type of reaction (see p. 137).

The local and general allergic reactions are caused by the Immediate or Type I mediated responses. The reactions responsible for the atypical clinical presentations are not yet fully known.

The diagnosis of insect stinging is usually obvious and no tests are required. Occasionally confirmatory tests may be required in an Allergy Clinic.

HOW TO AVOID INSECT STINGS

1. Do not let the child walk barefoot out-of-doors.
2. Avoid very bright and loose fitting clothing, because a bee might be attracted and trapped easily by it.
3. Wear dresses with long sleeves or jeans or stockings.
4. Do not use perfumes or scented soaps and cosmetics.
5. Avoid eating or drinking out-of-doors, e.g. ice creams, soft drinks.
6. Keep car windows shut when travelling in the countryside.
7. Keep insecticides readily available at home and in the car.

8. If the insect is near you or your child do not panic by making a
    lot of unnecessary gestures as these make the insect frightened.
    Remain still — as a rule the insect will fly away.

WHAT SHOULD YOU DO WHEN YOUR CHILD IS STUNG?

If you have tweezers or a fine knife remove the sting immediately.
Attempts at removal of a sting with your fingers are useless — you
will push it deeper into the skin and cause a longer reaction.

If the sting is inside the mouth, try to remove if you can but do
not spend time on it — take your child to the nearest Accident
and Emergency Department and tell the doctor or nurse what
happened. The reason for this action is that at times a very severe
swelling may occur within the mouth and obstruct the child's
breathing and swallowing — or even a more general reaction may
occur.

If you happen to have antihistamine tablets or syrup with you
give the child a first dose.

If your child has had a previous bee sting reaction then:

1. Obtain an adrenaline kit from your doctor — and know how to
    use it.
2. Keep antihistamines. Ensure these are readily available —
    keep them in your handbag! Have another set at home.
3. If your child has had a general reaction s/he will benefit from
    venom immunotherapy. Ask your doctor to refer you to an
    Allergy Clinic for assessment.

Chapter 14

Reactions to Drugs and Medications

A child may develop an adverse reaction to a drug or a medication which was prescribed for him/her in the course of an illness. These adverse reactions may mimic very closely an allergic response. Thus an adverse drug reaction may be due to:

- a toxic effect of the drug (most common)
- an allergic-like reaction — this occurs when a particular drug is given for certain conditions, e.g. if ampicillin is given to a child with glandular fever various rashes may occur.
- a true allergic reaction.
- co-incidental effect, i.e. with the medication administration, for instance, when the rash of measles may appear while the child is being given an antibiotic for an ear infection.

ALLERGIC DRUG REACTIONS

At the beginning of the twentieth century the use of antitoxins from horse serum was introduced into medicine. Serum sickness was the commonest general reaction to the horse serum. With the advent of synthetic drugs in the 1930s a plethora of adverse-drug reactions started to be reported from all over the world.

In general children with the common types of allergies do not develop adverse reactions to drugs more often than non-allergic children. Possibly allergy to aspirin and penicillin is a little more common in children with allergies.

About 2 in every 1,000 children admitted to hospital for some form of drug treatment will develop an adverse reaction to the drug or the combination of the drugs; of these reactions, about 5-8 per cent are due to true drug allergy.

HOW TO SUSPECT ALLERGIC DRUG REACTION

- the child has been treated with the same drug in the past and did not develop any reactions.
- the adverse reaction occurs during the course of the drug treatment or after many days treatment if this is the first exposure of the child to the drug.
- the beneficial effects of the drug are not known to be accompanied by such reactions.

WHAT TO DO IF YOU SUSPECT A DRUG REACTION

Stop giving any drugs to the child and inform your doctor *immediately* as some of these reactions can be very severe and life-threatening. If the child's condition appears to be deteriorating rapidly, bring him/her to the Accident and Casualty Department of your nearest hospital *at once* because the child may require emergency treatment.

The allergic drug reactions are the Immediate Type I or IgE mediated responses (see pp. 24-5), so that when the drug derived 'allergen' reacts with the specific IgE antibody, which is fixed to cells such as the mast cells or basophils, a reaction occurs causing the release of very potent pharmacological agents and thus clinical effects.

There are many types of allergic reaction. The most common are:

Anaphylaxis
A very serious generalized sensitivity to an allergen.

Urticaria (See p. 78)
May occur as a part of anaphylaxis or serum sickness. It is most common after antibiotics, some drugs used for epilepsy and tranquillizers.

Serum sickness

May occur within a few hours of taking the drug or as long as two or even three weeks after the drug was taken. The child may develop swelling of joints or fever or the kidneys may even become affected so that you may notice some blood in the urine. The most common drugs that cause a reaction are: some antibiotics, aspirin, and of course foreign serum.

There are many other reactions to drugs. Two of the common ones are:

Skin rashes

All sorts, from general redness of the skin to a 'measles'-like rash. In general these rashes have a tendency to cause itching as well. Antibiotics are common culprits. Occasionally a child will develop a skin rash when he is exposed to strong sunlight while taking a drug. Some soaps and cosmetics contain antiseptic agents which may act as the sensitizing substances.

Drug fever

No other allergic manifestations but recurrent fever. If you suspect this, discuss with your doctor because there are many other important causes of fever in young children.

> *Eric, aged 6 years, developed a 'cold', but since it did not go away in a few days time, his mother took him to the doctor who prescribed penicillin. Eric had had various antibiotics in the past without any problems. However, on the fourth day of taking penicillin, he became very feverish, rather miserable and soon afterwards he developed an intense 'red' rash all over his body which progressed within minutes to blisters. Some of these blisters were quite large and became easily damaged by rubbing them to relieve discomfort. Since in addition Eric refused to eat or drink he was admitted to hospital for further management.*

Comment: Eric became allergic to penicillin and produced clinically what is called by some doctors the Scalded Skin Syndrome 'because the rash and its blisters look like a scalded skin' (it is also termed Toxic Epidermal Necrolysis — a descriptive term). Sometimes this condition is caused by bacteria. The most common sensitivity substances are some antibiotics and some drugs for the treatment of epilepsy.

Eric recovered fully in ten days. He now carries a card stating that he is allergic to penicillin and similar antibiotics — this is most important because, if he were to be given penicillin inadvertently again, severe and life-threatening reaction could occur.

Glossary

The majority of terms are defined in the text and in the corresponding sections of the book.

The following is a general list:

Allergen A special substance, usually a protein molecule, causing an allergic reaction.

Allergy A term synonymous with hyper-sensitivity and which describes the different reactions mediated through immunological mechanisms. Some authorities limit the term to those reactions which are IgE mediated only.

Anaphylaxis A severe and generalized reaction to an agent to which the child has been exposed previously. Some reactions are non-immunologically mediated, i.e. mechanisms remain unknown.

Antibody A specific protein, i.e. immunoglobulin, produced in response to the stimulation by an antigen and being capable of reacting in a specific way with that particular antigen.

Antigen A substance which stimulates a specific immunological reaction.

Antitoxin An antibody that neutralizes a toxin which is a substance produced by micro-organisms.

Antihistamine A drug that counteracts the effects of histamine.

Atopy A inherited tendency to produce IgE induced reactions.

Auto-immunity	A state of immunological reactivity against 'own or self' antigens. Hence auto-immune diseases are the manifestations.
Basophil	A white blood cell that like the mast cell can be involved in allergic reactions.
Cell mediated immunity	A state of cell resistance, e.g. delayed type of hypersensitivity.
Complement	A system of specialized proteins in the serum which are required for the death of antigens when the antibody is present.
Cross-reaction	Reaction of the antibody with an antigen other than the homologous one — this implies that antigens are similar structurally.
Eosinophil	A white blood cell found often at the site of an allergic reaction. Its role in allergy remains unclear.
Histamine	One of the many pharmacological mediators released during an allergic reaction.
Idiosyncrasy	An abnormal reaction of a particular individual to a specific food, drug or other substance.
Immunity	The ability to react with antigen substances.
Immunogen	A substance producing immunity.
Immunoglobulins	A general name for the specialized proteins which possess antibody activity. They are related in structure.
Lymphocyte	A white cell of which there are two types, the B-cell and the T-cell. These cells are formed in the lymphoid tissues.
Lymphokines	Factors produced by stimulation of T-lymphocytes. They mediate T-cell functions and type of hypersensitivity.
Macrophage	A type of cell involved in engulfing micro-organisms, foreign substances or other cells.
Mast cell	A tissue cell involved in allergic reaction.

Placebo   A inactive substance.

Radioimmunoassay A method of quantifying the concentrations
                       of antibodies or allergens by using reagents that
                       have been labelled radioactively.

Reagin   The antibody of the IgE type which has the
                       ability to attach to cells in membranes or skin.

Thymus   A glandular organ of vertebrate animals
                       situated below the thyroid gland in the neck. It
                       produces lymphocytes in the very young to
                       influence immunological reactions. It shrinks
                       with age (from Greek 'thumos' — sweetbread).

Index

Abdominal colic, 49–50
Acupuncture, 123
Additives, food allergy and, 57–65
Adenoids
    and allergy, 92
    and surgery, 92
Adrenaline kit, 134
Allergens, 12
Allergy
    causes, 12–9
    history of, 9–11
    incidence, 31, 105
    miscellaneous, 35, 36
    prevention of, 36–8
    risk of, 29–30, 35
Anaphylaxis, 133
    and drugs, 128–9, 135–8
    treatment, 130
Animal epithelium, 16, 19
Antihistamines
    use of, 89
Aspirin sensitivity, 79, 100
Asthma
    allergic factors, 100
    definition, 100, 102–4
    diagnosis, 109
    IgE, 102–3
    incidence, 34, 105
    mechanism, 100-2
    mortality, 105
    prognosis, 105
    tests, 107–10
    treatment, 110–14, 115–17
Asthma Society, 110
Atopic dermatitis
    antihistamines, 74
    clinical features, 67–70
    diagnosis, 70
    incidence, 66–7
    treatment, 70–6
Atopy, 10
A20 dyes, 60–1

Basophils, 22
B-cells, 21, 22
Bathing and skin, 71
Bed-wetting and allergy, 65
Benzoates (see preservatives)
Bites and stings, 131–4
Breathing exercises and asthma, 121–2
Breast feeding and allergy, 14
Bronchial challenge, 109
Bronchodilators, 110–11

Cat dander, 16
Chest deformities and asthma, 122
Chocolate and headache, 41
    and coffee, 62
    and colic, 41
Coeliac Disease, 51
Conjunctivitis
    allergic, 98–9
    causes, 97
    treatment, 99–100
Contact dermatitis
    allergic, 77
    irritant, 77
    treatment, 78
Contactants, 77
Cosmetics, 77
Cow's milk
    clinical features, 12–13, 42, 47–88
    diagnosis, 47–8
    treatment, 49, 76
Cross-reactions, 12, 15

Dander, 16–17
Degranulation, 24–5
Deafness and allergy, 93, 95
Diet
    elimination, 45, 46, 76
    K–P, 61
Dog dander, 16
Drug allergy, 35

Ear, allergy of
    atopic dermatitis, 93–6
    contact dermatitis, 93
    inner ear, 96
Eczema, (see atopic dermatitis)
Egg sensitivity, 14
Environment and allergy, 29–30
Eyes, allergy of, 97–9
Exercise test and asthma, 100, 106–7
    and anaphylaxis, 129

Face, in allergy, 83
Feathers, 16
Fish allergy, 32
Food and allergy, 31–2, 39–65
Food colouring, 57
Food intolerance, 39
Food reactions, 40
    symptoms, 42

Games, effects of, 100, 106–7
Gastrointestinal allergy, 39–45
Grass pollens, 16–17

Hay fever, (see rhinitis)
Herbs, remedies of, 124
Heredity, 29
Histamine, 25–6
Homeopathy, 123–4
House dust, 19
House dust-mite, 19
Hyperactive child, 52–6
Hypersensitivity reactions,
    (see types of allergic reactions)
Hyperventilation and asthma, 104
Hypnotherapy, 124–5
Hyposensitization, 62, 72, 90–1

IgE and allergy, 24–5
Immunity, 20–23
Immunoglobulins, 22
Ingestants, 12
Inhalant allergy, 16–19
Injectants, 12
Insect allergy, 35
Irritable Bowel Syndrome, 50–1

Kidneys and allergy, (see bed-wetting)

Lungs and allergy, 101–2
Lung function tests, 107–8
Lymphokines, 21

Mast cell
    in allergy, 9–10, 24–6
    effects of drugs, 117–18
Migraine, 63–4
Milk allergy, (see cow's milk)
Milk proteins, 14
Monosodium glutamate, 59

Nose, allergy of, 34, 81–93
    immunotherapy, 90
    (see also hyposensitization
Nebuhaler, 117
Nebulizer, 111–12
Nervous system and allergy, 58–63

Occupational agents and asthma, 126–7
Otitis, (see ear)
Oxygen, in asthma, 103–4

Particles, allergens, 12, 18, 77
    of nebulized drugs, 111–12
Peak Expiratory Flow Meter, 107, 108
Penicillin allergy, 79
Photo allergy, 79

Physiology of asthma, 100–4
Polyps, 87
Preservatives, 57
Proctitis, allergic, 51
Prognosis, of allergy, 30
Psychological factors, 79, 100

Radioallergosorbent (RAST)
    in diagnosis, 45, 85
Rhinitis
    causes, 82–4
    treatment, 87–92

School attendance and asthma, 125
    and skin allergy, 71–2
Serum sickness, 137
Skin allergy
    causes, 33–4, 70
    features, 67–70
    tests, 85
    treatment, 70–6
Smoking, 37–8
Sodium cromoglycate, 89, 117–19
Steroids
    aerosols, 89, 119–20
Stings (see bites and stings)

Tar, coal, 74
Tartrazine, 60-1
T–cell, 21–5
Tension–Fatigue Syndrome, 51–3
Trees, pollens of, 19
Theophylline preparations, 120–1
Tonsillectomy and allergy, 92
Types of allergic reactions
    I, 24
    II, 26–7
    III, 26–7
    IV, 28

Urticaria
    causes, 78–9
    treatment, 80

Ventolin, 111
Vernal conjunctivitis, 98–9
Virus infections and asthma, 100

Wheat, 12, 15, 41

Yeast, 19, 41

Xanthines, (see Theophylline)